When Spirits
Lie;
Living with F.A.S.D.

L. ELIZABETH BAKER

ISBN 978-1-954345-58-4 (paperback)
ISBN 978-1-954345-59-1 (digital)

Rushmore Press LLC
1 800 460 9188
www.rushmorepress.com

Printed in the United States of America

Preface

I MET ELIZABETH LATE 2016 when I was searching for a service dog for my son, who was diagnosed with autism at a young age.

I did not know at the time that not only would I find the perfect dog, but that I'd also learn of an incredible life story.

As our cooperation and friendship grew, I began to feel that I had met an extraordinary person. When she asked me to read the manuscript for her book, that feeling was soon confirmed.

When I began to read her story, it was during the height of the COVID19 pandemic in Canada. As a physician working both in a family medicine clinic and a rural hospital, it was understandably quite a stressful time for me. I read Elizabeth's book during those rare periods of respite, taking in the multifaceted story as I went along.

This book delves into the perspective of someone living with Fetal Alcohol Syndrome, and brilliantly characterizes the unique joys and challenges that it may bring. It also highlights society's poor understanding and lack of awareness of a condition with which roughly four percent of the Canadian population lives with.

This book is an emotionally charged rollercoaster as we are taken through each chapter of her fascinating life- from age four all the way through adulthood. The message of this book is a powerful one. We see one woman's resilience and a thirst for survival at any cost, and just how far determination can take us in life.

They say that each life story is a novel, and after reading this book I learned another life story worth telling. I feel very fortunate to have met Elizabeth, and privileged to share my experience with her.

To my family, she has given us the gift of a wonderful service dog that has changed our lives for the better.

To you, the reader, she will give a heartfelt story about the strength of the human spirit.

Dr. Agron Alija
London, ON

Foreword

By
Doris J. Baker, B.Sc., M.S.W.

— • ● ● ○ ● ● • —

As you pause and think about it, there are many ways a family is created. This book will ask you to consider that fact. Another fact is that many children are damaged, in a variety of ways, before they are born. Facts also establish that many children are hurt and damaged after birth.

This narrative deals with such factors and urge each reader to take personal responsibility to not damage a child. Fetal Alcohol Spectrum Disorder (FASD) does not have to be the diagnosis of any more children. The information is mounting that both egg and sperm need to be protected from the damage from alcohol ingestion.

The heroine of this narrative is now a middle-aged woman who has developed coping skills and a desire to assist others who are FASD survivors and to prevent others from being so diagnosed.

Our survivor heroine began life as another baby born to an alcoholic woman, was in and out of care with the Children's Aid Society until she was made a ward of the crown and available for adoption. Her time in a Foster home as a toddler, resulted in sexual molestation by the foster father. In this home, she had few toys, simple foods and lots of admonition re: not being a good girl. When she was nearly five, we met. She was to have a forever family and my husband and I had room in our hearts for another child.

The usual preparations and legal measures were all done and at five she moved into our home with a new brother, father and mother. This was a time of many challenges for each family member. The information supplied by C.A.S. was brief, inaccurate and somewhat creative!

Her school years resulted in many challenges, uncertainties and poor behavioral choices. Some became known to us and others were hidden. She struggled to allow herself to be integrated into our family and to accept the talents and abilities she had. For example, she earned considerable recognition for her musical skills and abilities but always wondered if such acknowledgements were real. As such, she set them aside.

Compassion for others is a central element of her life. She is a great Mother to her two children and has been in a successful relationship for over 15 years. She has established a successful business and reputation.

She is our daughter. She has F.A.S.D.

When Spirits Lie

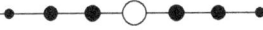

———— • • • ○ • • • ————

As THE OWNER AND DIRECTOR of my Service Dog training facility, I often find myself either on a plane or on the road delivering various dogs to their new homes, followed by a week of training with myself and the client. I had again packed my car the night before yet another trip and planned to leave early the next morning with another dog to deliver to anxiously awaiting clients. The dog was ready and yet I felt the familiar pang of sadness as I prepared to say goodbye to yet another one of my babies. Each dog I have said goodbye to is my baby first before I pass them off to the new client to help them in their daily lives and strive for independence. Maxine (Max) knew something was up the next morning as I arose early from my bed and prepared for the long trip. I let her outside to relieve herself and have some fresh air before loading her into the car. Although we had gone for rides a hundred times before, this time, she didn't want to get into the car right away and I had to coax her in. When she finally jumped in, I patted her a few more times and told her she was going to have a wonderful life with her new family. I climbed into my car behind the wheel and started the car up as Max laid down in the back with a sigh. Our journey began uneventfully and after hours of driving, I was only a couple hours from my destination. I stopped to let Max out so she could stretch her legs and have a drink of water while I ate my lunch, I had prepared that morning. I watched as she sniffed the different smells in the air and inspected each tree within reach. She looked at me eating and tried to convince me she needed a bite too with the cutest puppy eyes she could muster. I swore her to secrecy as I gave her some bread with a little peanut butter on it and she happily gobbled it down. I reloaded her into the car after we played for a little while and continued on our journey. I was driving down a familiar stretch of highway thinking about my beautiful white shepherd I was delivering to the client. I hoped my week spent training both the client and the dog together as a team would go smoothly, as we accomplished a list of training exercises that would be required before I could leave them. I mentally made my list of tasks to accomplish as I drove and I was in a good mood, enjoying the spring sunshine and the scenery as I approached a familiar town. It was the town I was born in and spent the first four tumultuous years of my life. I had travelled this route many times before and knew it well, but I never had the desire to stop and look around. My mind wandered as I read the familiar signs and continued on my journey.

I found myself wondering if I could even find the foster home I lived in prior to my adoption and whether or not I really wanted to find it. I could picture it in my mind, the two-storey white farm house at the end of a gravel driveway bordered by a wire fence, with the grey weathered barn off to the right of the house. The large green pasture in front of the barn where the cows grazed lazily in the summer sun and the woods behind the house, beyond the back pasture. I immediately felt a sudden sense of dread. It took me by surprise after all these years, that I should feel this way; I was an adult, a mother, I owned my own successful business and had built a good reputation that I had spent years cultivating. After all, there really wasn't any reason I should feel this way, the people involved were now deceased and couldn't hurt me anymore. But still…the feeling persistently, stubbornly remained.

I tried to push the thoughts from my mind as I continued on my journey and forced myself to think about the days to come. I eventually arrived at my destination and dropped Max off at the clients. After a short meeting with the family, I left her with her new family. She cried a little as I left. I felt that familiar ache in my tummy as I walked away from yet another one of my babies and continued on to my hotel to check in. My room was adequate, just another hotel room really, I had been in so many doing this job and knew the general set up before I even entered. I ordered in dinner and pulled out my laptop to begin looking at maps of the area out of unintended curiosity. I wasn't exactly sure of what I was looking for or even why, but eventually found myself looking at the town map of where I had once lived. I Googled a map from 1969 as well as the foster family I had stayed with and looked for land marks I might recognize. After searching, I found one landmark that seemed somewhat familiar. It startled me that I actually found it and I took note of the roads around the landmark. One of them was the road I lived on for a short, but traumatic time, but which one? I didn't know for sure, but thought perhaps on my way home, I might just take a look. What could it hurt? I tried to change my attention to the television as I settled in to sleep. Unfortunately, I didn't sleep well that night as the nightmares flooded back and I tossed and turned, at one point waking up screaming.

I continued with my work during the rest of the week training the client and Max to work together as a team. We worked in shopping malls, department stores, the school and even restaurants as they learned to work together as a well-trained team. On the final day, I spoke with the family and gave Max a quick pat goodbye before leaving her forever. They were happy with their service dog and the client was anticipating a new found independence which I encouraged. As I pulled away for the last time, I had my usual little cry after saying goodbye to yet another great dog.

I had been sleeping poorly all week although I had never given the client any indication of how distracted I was. I hoped this last night I would sleep well before the long drive home. Saturday morning finally arrived, I checked out of the hotel and packed up my car. I stopped for gasoline and a muffin before I continued on my way, this time taking the back roads towards the little town I remembered.

Yet another beautiful day for travelling and I enjoyed the many different lakes that dotted the rocky landscape covered with endless patches of forest and moose caution signs every few miles. I wistfully thought of stopping to do some fishing, but pressed on in my journey, half aware that I seemed to be on a mission. After driving for a couple hours, I began to realize that the scenery was starting to look familiar. I am really not sure how I ended up on the particular road I found myself driving on and don't really remember turning, but I must have somewhere along the way. A few more miles along and I came to a bend to the right in the road ahead and my stomach went into knots. As I rounded the bend, there it was. The house. The barn. The driveway and the pasture. With a surprised gasp, I slowed down my car and then pulled over to the side of the road. Everything was as I remembered it. Some trees were missing and others were much bigger, but it was The House I had lived in prior to being adopted. I stared at the scene for a few moments before I opened my car door and got out. I began walking along the shoulder of the road, hearing the gravel crunch beneath my feet with each step. Everything seemed to be happening in slow motion as I was looking at the yard, the house, the porch and my eyes rose to the upstairs window where my bedroom would have been and then the wave hit me. I was suddenly assaulted with overwhelming nausea that I had absolutely no control over and I threw myself forward while I began to vomit. Gut wrenching, unending waves, over and over as though I was expelling some demon that had suddenly possessed me. My stomach protested violently to the onslaught of pain and anguish that overwhelmed me. When the waves finally subsided, I was embarrassed and hopeful no one saw me, as I quickly made my way back to my car. I sat in my car feeling stunned by what had just happened and found myself exhausted from the extreme purge of emotions.

I took one last look, then started my car again and began to drive away. I was in a state of shock that I had actually found the place and I was emotionally fragmented between wanting to weep in pain and scream from rage. So many emotions were fighting for dominance within me that I was confused and knew I needed to pull myself together. I drove my car into the little town and found a parking lot to pull into that had some trees that would provide shade, off in a back corner. I hid my car beneath the trees, turned the engine off and began to weep uncontrollably. I wept deeply with such sorrow mixed with anger, confusion and disbelief, that I sat there for sometime before I could pull myself together. After some time, I texted my daughter and told her I was going to pull over and take a nap, as I was feeling sleepy. I often kept in touch with her when I was on the road and often, she would talk to me and help keep me awake and alert.

This time I couldn't talk, nor did I think she would understand my turmoil and I decided I would try to have a nap. The house was clearly in my head and hard as I tried, I couldn't think of anything else, but I was so exhausted I fell asleep anyways. I awoke with a start two hours later, rolled down my window and shakily lit a cigarette. I couldn't believe what I had experienced and how it badly it had affected me after all these years. All the memories I thought I had deeply buried, all the emotions I thought I had dealt with were really still there, just below the surface and I felt like an immense failure, a fraud. I hadn't moved on at all, I was still that frightened little girl who had been abused, neglected and tortured. I had accomplished nothing and was still being haunted by my memories.

I wanted, no desperately needed to talk to my mother. I knew she would help me think this awful experience through, because at that moment I was simply reacting. I wasn't thinking clearly and had no idea where to go from there or how to organize my thoughts. I was an emotional mess and needed some kind of direction in the midst of the turmoil that was engulfing me. I grabbed my cell phone and texted my daughter to let her know I was on the road again and then turned on my car and began driving the long drive home. I arrived after dark and following brief conversations with my family, I went to my bedroom and called my mother. I began to cry as I told her in detail of my appalling experience and she quietly listened. Finally, I finished my narrative and there was a short silence on the phone followed by my wonderful, understanding mother saying to me lovingly, "Congratulations, it's about time!"

My Secret

———— • • • ○ • • • ————

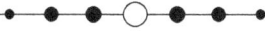

I HAVE LIVED WITH MY secret for over 50 years, fiercely trying to guard it protectively, as though it were a shameful, obscene truth that must never be released. I have had relationships, friends, lovers and a husband without them knowing my dark secret. I have had two beautiful, physically healthy children, been a loving and involved mother and yet did not share my secret with my children until they were older. It took months of wrestling with my shame, while trying to find courage and faith in my relationship to finally tell my current partner. I have lived in my community amongst neighbors and friends who never had a clue. I have developed a thriving business, a healthy reputation and respect in my field amongst my colleagues, without anyone knowing. I have been so very careful not to divulge any part of my secret…until now.

My shame was cultivated and protected by a 'don't tell' reaction I have learned from societies response over the years. It was suggested by those who did know my secret that informing others could result in my being seen as less capable, as if I might suddenly revert to idiocy. It could diminish my standing in the community to the extent that I would no longer be taken seriously, as if I were suddenly to lose a great portion of my brain and be incapable of intelligent thought. I could be immediately seen as brain injured, perhaps intellectually disabled or at the very least mentally incapable and I couldn't stand the thought of the potential piteous stares as I divulged my secret.

My secret is far from being of my own doing, it was in fact inflicted upon me. Regardless, this does not seem to lessen the stigma associated with it being made known. I have wrestled for years with whether it was wise to make my secret public knowledge and the decision was not easily arrived at. I involved my family in the process, knowing it would affect their lives as well, they have offered me nothing but support. I know I will lose acquaintances and perhaps even business based upon this secret becoming public knowledge and I am now prepared to accept this loss of respect as well as possible revenue.

I don't appear different, in fact I was perceived as attractive in my younger years, intelligent and very professional. I am seen by some physicians as 'disabled' and others as a 'miracle', but after hearing this term from a friend, consider myself 'differently-abled'. Yes, I am challenged on a daily basis, however I have learned coping strategies to manage the variety of issues I encounter. I have also learned countless excuses that can buy me others indulgence in a pinch.

My memory is affected, but I have taught myself simple 'cheats' to bypass questions. Much like an illiterate individual uses the excuse of having lost his or her glasses; I can say I had a momentary lapse and laugh it off. People assume sometimes correctly that I am very busy and perhaps distracted, which frequently works in my favor. My multiple physical and health issues can be disguised as 'getting older' or having pulled a muscle or from being overweight. No one ever looks closely enough to notice the subtle differences, quirks or behaviors I might have. The societal attitude of 'personal space' most definitely works in my favor and I simply increase my space a little more than others. I never allow many people to be too close.

When the cause of my condition is broached, people tend to change the subject quickly, look away or are visibly uncomfortable. There are misguided apologies, excuses given as to why it shouldn't - but might happen in this day and age; although the same knowledge of its affects was known almost fifty years ago. To say it is a completely preventable condition is at best naïve and at worst dismissive. It is the equivalent of an opinion when it's about someone else, but when it becomes personal, or they find out about your diagnosis, they become appalled, indignant or even enraged. But what good does this do when the damage has already been done?

I have come to terms with my diagnosis long ago and experienced the prescribed stages of grief, without it progressing my understanding of myself or my condition whatsoever. I have spent years being enraged and wanting revenge to no avail; it has not assisted in my daily existence one bit. I have meticulously researched my diagnosis almost to the point of expertise and still am left with infinite questions. So, what am I left with other than my anger and resentment? To live, experience and inform, that is all I can do.

Society is not prepared to handle my diagnosis, let alone comprehend all the symptomology and psychology linked to it. There is an additional societal 'There but by the grace of God' belief as many pregnancies are unplanned or initially unknown. Behaviors associated with my diagnosis are minimally understood and generally undervalued by educators, parents and physicians, seen simply as excuses when, in reality they are far from it. Those of us in the world with this diagnosis genuinely wish for better understanding, not only from others but for ourselves. Physicians are inclined to giving a morbid prognosis, leaning towards institutionalization at some point in our lives, whether from drug addiction, psychiatric illness or legal misdeeds. We are subject to significantly higher incidences of addiction, suicide and violence with little or no hope given in comfort. Statistics are spewed out in what seem random convulsions, with no personal link to ourselves, and we are left to wonder 'so whose projected outcome should I follow today?' Our futures are bleak, so 'they' say and again I wonder who the hell 'they' are and why have 'they' decided this for me? What about what I want?

I want to say perhaps I'll be a Doctor or a Lawyer, but I know the statistics, so I decide perhaps it's best not to try. I could be a famous musician, but I am prone to addiction, so perhaps this is not a good choice. Maybe a rocket scientist, but I have multiple learning disabilities…maybe, again no. I am given so many arguments against choices I wish to pursue I just want to scream.

Many of my fellow 'diagnosed' and I have come from difficult or even traumatic backgrounds having been in the care of Children's Aide Societies, foster homes and etc. We have received little or no medical history from Children's Aide to add to the ever-expanding file on our physician's desk and are met with the polite response of 'Oh, I see' when asked. I have yet to have a physician maintain eye contact with me when I inform them of my history, as though they share some personal shame. Our parents who have adopted their pretty little girl or cute little boy have been given very little warning of the difficulties they might face in our rearing. They too are given the diagnosis, symptoms and statistics, leaving them wondering what on earth they have gotten themselves into, if they decide to continue with the adoption process at all. The idea of passing on some semblance of hope is a foreign doctrine to many physicians and this same doctrine also prohibits positive thinking. The worst-case scenario is always in the foreground of every discussion and the black hole of diagnosis just keeps getting deeper and darker.

Some adoptive families decide against adopting due to the lack of any positive encouragement and the child is left to grow up in the system to 'age out'. This means numerous foster homes, potential juvenile facilities and then, at age 18, they can be unceremoniously ushered to the proverbial curb. Parents who do choose to continue on the adoption path must be very special indeed and most certainly require extreme patience, patience and more patience! They will undoubtedly receive little to no support from government, agencies, educators or Physicians, as we age and the school system is the least informed to the point of negligence at best. It's not that the information is unknown or unattainable; it's simply that educators believe this is an excuse and refuse to acknowledge this diagnosis in many parts of the world. All the studies have yet to find their way to be digested during teachers' conferences or schools and remarkably many teachers I have spoken to know more about Autism than FASD. I find this to be shameful, however who is to blame for the lack of knowledge being released? Until governments understand how much money they are spending on children with FASD through the legal and medical establishments, the lack of understanding will prevail.

We are a challenge, an enigma that constantly changes between individuals. The studies conducted project more information that joins a vast wasteland of information that might or might not pertain to your child. No two of us are identical and the enormity of it all is frustrating. Children who are adopted at a later age may have additional abuse or trauma included into the mix which only serves to add exponentially to the difficulties the family will face. Then we have baggage that can range from mild to extreme and could include neglect, sexual abuse, witnessing violence, extreme neglect or even abandonment. With our diagnosis, emotions are difficult enough, but then to add these lovely additions including a delay to mature to the still growing list, it's a wonder we survive at all. Many of us who do survive are left to remember those who did not.

The diagnosed child is a contradiction in terms, in that we are expected to learn by society, family and educators, but not expected to succeed by social and medical statistics. Society outwardly observes us as 'normal' unless there are clear facial or physical indications. The 'normal' almost attractive features we are born with are an additional malicious curse; people expect more from attractive individuals and become almost incensed when this does not occur. Attractive people are expected to excel in society, be socially dynamic, intelligent and prosperous. They are expected to hold down executive, white collar jobs with status, family and friends oozing from their pores.

This exacerbates an already delicate anxiety level that causes us to become even more apprehensive and self-deprecating. We self-condemn and berate as punishment for our crimes of possessing multiple learning disabilities and our inability to be social. We can snap an unwarranted retort just as well as the next person on a bad day, but we back it up with additional resentment, anger and confusion. Often, we know we are being unreasonable, but simply can't stop the rage in the moment. It took me years to learn to walk away from an argument and I still have great difficulty in performing this simple, yet harrowing task. We have great difficulty organizing our numerous and conflicting thoughts, let alone our sock drawer, but in the next instance we are performing wondrous works of music or painting a magnificent work of art. We are, at times, a demonstration of irony in its truest form.

I fight with emotional turmoil every day and constantly wonder if I'm doing or saying the right thing. I am obsessed with presenting a professional front but I am full of insecurity and a fear of rejection. I am over 50 years old and still fear my parents giving up on me. For most of my adolescence and teen years I tried to make this very fear become reality and yet, they are still here, supporting and loving me. 'Ah well, maybe tomorrow' my mother will tease me with a smile. And yet tomorrow comes and goes, and they are still here. Such incredible people they are!

I have decided my partner in life is a saint, though I'm quite sure the church won't accept him. His miraculous deed is simply living with me day after day, yet to me it is miraculous. He loves me and this concept after 15 years is still so foreign to me. I know I trust him and love him, but I still wonder if I truly understand that kind of love. I love my children and know they love me too. This kind of love, I understand, I know I would die for them without a thought for myself. There is nothing they could ever do that would cause me to stop loving them, I am fiercely sure!

What is my dark, shameful secret? I am living with Fetal Alcohol Spectrum Disorder.

The Child

I DECIDED TO WRITE THIS book after speaking and working with so many parents of children with F.A.S.D. and being asked to pass on information not given by psychiatrists, psychologists, specialists, doctors and social workers, etc. I have been begged on occasions to 'translate' for their children's behavior, being at a complete loss of why Jr. did this or said that. The questions of 'How does it feel when? 'or 'What is he thinking when?' are only scratching the surface of the parents' unlimited questions in their search to understand a most unusual child. Furthermore, trying to explain that while many symptoms are similar, one would be hard pressed to find two identical children! Having a unique insight inside this world by someone who has Fetal Alcohol Spectrum Disorder has led parents to inundate me with requests of assistance in helping to unlock the mysteries so that they might understand their child. As a person with F.A.S.D., we do not necessarily read the textbooks or the latest literature spewed out by professionals with varying university degrees. Instead we live it daily, experience every nuance associated with it, and lose so very much in our lives because of it. I am not here to provide diagrams, graphs, or the latest statistics. I am here to try to describe, to the best of my ability, how it feels, how it affects and how it dominates one's life on a daily basis. I am here to define how we need to compromise, adjust and eliminate certain expectations in our lives in order to cope with this damage. I will try to explain our behavior, our thinking patterns, our coping mechanisms and our way of life. I will try not to judge, cry, or rant. I promise nothing but an inside view of life with F.A.S.D. and so I must start at the beginning. The first thing you must understand above and beyond anything else is that this is brain DAMAGE. This damage is beyond repair and will never nor can ever be 'fixed' or cured so please stop trying. We can learn coping skills, new learning techniques or cheats to get around some of the damage, but it is never going to go away.

I have to say that this desire to 'fix' is our biggest curse in life. Parents try initially but then it's the teachers who take up the rallying cry. My biggest antagonists in my life have been well meaning teachers, who simply did not get it, or want to understand this is brain damage we are talking about here. We are not lazy, stupid or defiant; we simply cannot be expected to learn at the same rate or pace as other children. It does not necessarily mean that I cannot learn, but I certainly am not able to in the parameters you or the ministry of education has prescribed for every child, nor do we fit in the Autism Spectrum section of the teaching manual. The sooner educators' figure this out, the sooner the violent outbursts and frustration will subside.

Once upon a time, there was a beautiful little princess who lived in a marvelous castle with her loving and doting parents, the king and queen. One day an evil troll kidnapped the poor princess and stole her away from her perfect life…

This is the story I imagined as a child. Otherwise I would have to accept the possibility that I was truly rejected by not only my biological 'mother' but 'father' as well. After all, rejection of a birth parent is the one ultimate betrayal that is so cruelly unthinkable. If my own 'parents' didn't want me, why would anyone else? This is a genuine issue for many adoptive children and becomes a commonality amongst us. Rejection was to become the biggest torment in my life as I would engage in exhaustive manipulation to prove I was not 'worth' acceptance. This is when I also began to entertain the notions that something might be wrong with me either intellectually or mentally. These notions continue to haunt me even now as I wonder if I am capable of accomplishing what I hope to. The real reason I was placed in care had absolutely nothing to do with me or my impairments. Instead it was due to the birth 'mother's' inability to care for me for various reasons. I honestly cannot answer whether it is better for a child to have known the biological parents or not, as I didn't know or remember mine before I was adopted. For the most part it seems to me to be a 'damned if you do damned if you don't' scenario. Either way, the baggage is there, it's just a matter of whom or what caused it.

I will explain here that because of what I learned of my biological 'family'; I prefer to call them donors. They never assumed the role of 'mother' or 'father' and I have chosen to protectively reserve those titles for the people who adopted, raised, loved and supported me. I have found over the years as I mature that I now fiercely guard this relationship between my parents and myself as never before, now that as a parent I truly understand how very incredible they are!

I was to learn that I was in fact rescued from a very neglectful and abusive situation. My biological, maternal donor had come from a respected family based in the military. As a teenager, she had rebelled and was an alcoholic, drug experimenting teen mother, with two children already. It was in the nineteen sixties, during the hippie craze of drug and alcohol experimentation and free love. I was the third of six, unplanned children altogether. I was removed from her custody approximately six months after birth and placed in the Children's Aide custody. I was found to have had cigarette burns on my body, a hand that had been burned by some sort of liquid, and was severely undernourished, amongst many other injuries and illnesses due to malnutrition and tuberculosis. I was described as 'a very quiet baby, who never made a sound'. I believe this should have been the first red flag regarding my development. At the time of removal from her care I was in an extremely soiled diaper and being 'cared' for by my siblings, who were both under the age of five years.

I was initially placed in the care of my elderly, biological great-grandparents who, after a short time, decided they were unable to care for me. It is my understanding that these people were wonderful individuals who tried very hard to take care of me, but simply couldn't manage the needs of an infant at their advanced age. I was again removed and placed in foster care after becoming a ward of the crown. In total, I experienced five consecutive placements until my last one at the age of four, which is not conducive to bonding. I now believe I also had attachment disorder, based on the thoughts and feelings I had growing up. I arrived at my last placement when I was four and I will remember it for the rest of my life. Here, I learned how to manipulate in order to simply survive. While I do know the protocols for being accepted as a foster parent today are quite intensive, along with criminal background checks etc., they weren't over forty years ago. In the grand scheme of life, I was there under a year, but it seemed like an eternity for me and one of my sisters.

I arrived at the "Smith' family farm and remember the little white, two storey house, barn and outhouse. The country was beautiful and emerald green with rocky open spaces where one might have thought I could run and be a child. The 'Smith' family consisted of Mr. and Mrs., as well as two biological children, both teenagers. The youngest was a teenage boy, the eldest was a girl, whom I don't recall being around that much. I was placed in this home with my biological eldest sister, by four years. My sister and I had our place within the family home, but we were kept outside the family itself, as though we were part of the furniture. We were just a means to an income, but more than that, an inconvenience. We were told repeatedly how lucky we were they took us in and cared for us, as no one wanted us. During celebrations and holidays, we were placed in the farthest corner, away from everything and everyone. We were not to participate in any way and were to remain quiet at all times. If we did not comply with the rules, Mr. had a two-foot-long strap made of double-folded stitched leather, which he would happily use. I can remember that strap as clearly as though it were sitting right in front of me, it was kept hanging on the wall of their kitchen like a trophy. We would wind up with red welts on our hands, backs or backsides, which would be there for days.

The days often began with terror over breakfast, when we were given our oatmeal. We were allowed to put brown sugar on it, but we had to finish all of it. If we didn't, our hands would be introduced to the strap. Many times, I would vomit out of fear and even to this day, I cannot eat breakfast first thing in the morning. Our daily diet consisted of Oatmeal, Bologna, mashed potatoes, fried chicken, peanut butter or brown sugar and butter sandwiches. I still cannot stomach bologna and don't much care for chicken either. Suffice to say I was malnourished, underweight and under height when I was finally adopted. All meals had to be fully finished before we could leave the table, or face yet another beating. We were constantly reminded of the fact we were taking food from our foster family and that we didn't deserve it. I have had difficulties with food control since then. My reward is food, and I can binge with the best of them

I still remember the look Mr. 'S.' would get on his face before he would reach for the strap. His eyes would open wide and his face get quite red then he would explode into a rage and we would both would start running. After a particularly severe episode of abuse, I remember my sister deciding to run away, with me toddling along behind. We weren't gone long, nor did we go far, but this also resulted in my sister being rather savagely beaten with the strap. We ended up being found by Mr. 'S' and he took us home and sat us at the kitchen table. He asked my sister why she ran away and didn't she appreciate all they had done for us. As soon as she began to speak, he grabbed my sister by the arm and dragged her over to where the strap hung on the wall. As he reached for it, she tried desperately to wriggle free but he had her arm in a vice -like grip. He brought down the strap on her leg with a terrible smack and she howled in pain. First the spot on her leg went white, then a deep angry red as it began to swell. He raised his hand and struck her twice more, once on the buttocks and once on her back before demanding that she and I go to our room without supper. Mrs. 'S' began to clear the table as she said in a reprimanding tone "You should've known better, I told you!" We made our way upstairs to our little 'room' on the landing as my sister sobbed. My sister laid gingerly on her lower bunkbed, whimpering in her bed as I tried to soothe her by rubbing her and she howled in pain. I never touched her again after a beating. I never wanted to hurt her like they had.

Another occasion I remember quite well was when the family went shopping and left me behind in the store. It was a Kmart style store with all the large display cabinets arranged neatly on the floor. I remember wandering around the store looking for my foster family but couldn't find them. I walked up and down the aisles and no one would even look at me when I did see someone. As the store cleared out and got quieter, I ended up crawling inside a square display cabinet when I was too afraid to look anymore. I spent the night there, behind the sliding doors. The store lights were turned off and it was dark and terrifying as I cried myself to sleep in the cabinet. The next morning, I was found crying and was returned to the 'Smith's'. No police were called, nor CAS to my knowledge. It was a different time with different rules I suppose, but I don't understand losing a child for an entire evening.

When I returned home with my foster parents, again I was sat at the kitchen table. This time, it was my turn for the strap and I began to cry. This just served to infuriate Mr. 'S' even more and he grabbed the strap and began swinging. He emphasized each strike with a word and he told me to "Never do that again!" Exactly four strikes of the strap, four large welts at various positions on my body, four times I screamed in pain. He then shoved me towards my room, where I was ignored until the next morning. Every time I moved on my bed, I whimpered in pain as quietly as I could. I remember being sore for a long time after that.

When experiencing the physical abuse, sometimes it would be with the strap, other times it would be a quick back hand across the face or buttocks which inevitably sent me flying across the room. One occasion I remember hitting the door frame, then being on the sofa as Mrs. 'S' said something about him hitting me too hard and him saying that I had 'pissed him off' and that 'the little shit deserved it!' Mrs. 'S' never tried to protect us or interfere in the abuse, nor did she participate in it except for verbally. She was never too busy to admonish us for being 'ugly' or undesired 'little bastards', as well as telling us no one would ever love us.

On several occasions an elderly woman my foster parents knew looked after me, while they went out. I would be driven to her home and she always wore a black dress with her white hair pulled tightly into a bun. She would take me into her house, which always smelled funny to me and she would place me in a little closet which she would then lock, for the duration until they returned for me. It was a dark little closet with not much room to move around, but I could see with a tiny bit of light under the locked door, that shone from the room on the other side. Sometimes I would sleep while other occasions, I would tell myself stories. One time I was in 'my' closet when a spider's eggs began to hatch. I didn't like spiders but had not developed my phobia until that day. I began to scream as hundreds of baby spiders crawled all over me and through my hair. The old woman told my foster parents that I spent the afternoon running and screaming through her house and that I couldn't come back; when in fact I had been beating the locked door with my now raw hands, trying to escape from the spiders. I am fine with large spiders such as tarantulas' and even enjoy holding them. It's the small ones that terrify me still and I often need assistance to get them away from me. The experience resulted in my acquiring this lifelong phobia, with paralyzing results. Fortunately, I have very understanding children who rescue me regularly. I remember hearing that the old lady in black had died and I also remember smiling all the way home in the back of the car; I was happy she was dead. I knew I would never see that closet again!

Night time at the 'Smith's' could be even worse and became a time of awful dread for both my sister and I. Most evenings we would watch country music shows and a star named Kitty Wells on television or the televangelist Billy Graham. My sister and I would then be ushered off to bed by Mrs. 'S'. We would put on our pajamas, crawl into bed as quietly as we could and pray under our breaths to go to sleep. Sometimes we would lay there and begin to hear Mr. 'Smith's' footsteps coming up the stairs. I would try to shrink into the farthest corner of my bed as we would await the horror we knew was about to follow. He would come to the top of the stairs and we could hear him breathing heavily from the climb as he removed the belt from his pants. He always took time deciding which one of us he would pick for his pleasure while we desperately tried to pretend, we were sound asleep. Inevitably he would make up his mind and pull one of us off our bed and he would remove our nighty or just pull it up. I never watched him abuse my sister, I just hid and stayed quiet so I wouldn't be next. When he chose me, he never had me face him, but would turn me around and begin to fondle me between my legs with one hand as he pleasured himself with the other. I tried to be as quiet as possible when he did this, but it hurt and I would often wince from the pain. He told me I liked it and that I was a dirty girl in a strange sounding voice and I never turned around until it was time for me to get back into bed. When I did, the back of my nighty was always soaked and I thought I had wet myself. I knew Mrs. 'S' would be very angry with me for wetting the bed and that I wouldn't get any food the next day as result, but that was ok as I was never really hungry after those nights. I remember one time he began as he normally did and I was standing in front of him as his fingers probed between my legs. He suddenly wrapped his hands around my arms and picked me up. He wrapped one arm around me as he grabbed himself again but this time, I felt something different go between my legs. It was bigger and hurt terribly as he 'bounced' me up and down on his lap and I screamed in pain. He put his hand over my mouth and wriggled under me a little more and then stopped. I felt like I had been ripped apart and I was bleeding from between my legs. He panicked when he saw the blood and picked me up and threw me on my upper bunk as my head hit the wall. I laid there weeping as he told me to shut up and he got dressed. He told me to keep my mouth shut and be down for breakfast in the morning and then left the landing. My sister waited for his footsteps to stop then she reached for a box of Kleenex and crawled up to my bunk. She spread my legs apart and began to wipe off the blood as she told me I would be ok. She told me he did that to her too and she knew how much it hurt but if he did it again, it wouldn't hurt as badly as the first time.

My foster brother tried on a couple occasions to fondle us as well but that's a far as it went with him. Either my sister or myself would endure these men whispering in our ears to 'shut up and don't move' while they occupied themselves. After one particularly brutal incident, I found out that my social worker was coming the next day for a surprise visit. I waited for her to arrive and then proceeded to inform her of what had occurred the previous evening. She listened intently and then told me everything would be fine. She gave me a pat on the head and told me to go outside and play for a while. She walked to the kitchen with me as I continued outside and she sat the table with my foster parents. She immediately told Mr. and Mrs. 'Smith' everything I had said and they, of course, denied everything.

After the Social Worker left, I was called into the kitchen and Mr. 'Smith' was standing there with his hand behind his back as he leaned against a chair. He asked me what I had told the Social Worker and I replied with a very frightened, quiet "nothing". He called me to come to him and I slowly walked towards him. When I stood in front of him, he told me to turn around and place my hands on the table. I did as he demanded and he raised his hand from behind his back and brough the strap down on my back again and again. I don't remember how many times he hit me with the strap, but I do remember Mrs. 'S' finally coming around the corner and telling him to stop; that I was no good dead.

I crawled up the stairs to my room and tried to climb into my bed. Even my sister was mad at me and she pushed me onto my bed, off of hers. I never spoke out again and it took me years to be able to finally say something to my mother. I learned to disconnect myself from the abuse while it was happening. I would lie there like a rag doll and disassociate from reality. It was just a matter of disappearing into my imagination. Over time, my pain threshold grew and I began to be able to tolerate almost anything. Eventually anytime he used the strap, I would barely flinch and not make any sound at all.

There were many other instances of abuse I might account, but I believe you have the idea of the brutality we experienced. I also need to protect myself here, when I do discuss my abuse, I often have nightmares for weeks and I do not wish to lose anymore sleep over the memories.

As far as I understood at the tender age of four, I was home. This foster family was my permanent family and I had accepted this as fact. I did my best to exist without being noticed or draw attention to myself and often played outside amidst the farm animals and fields. I loved the animals and thoroughly enjoyed being with them. I felt they understood me and me, them. They were gentle and kind with me, even the cattle, when no human was. I first learned about tenderness from a cow that would gently nudge grass out of my hand and push me gently for more. I adored the huge drooly creatures and never feared them, nor them me. I walked the fields with them and pick little yellow flowers while I daydreamed. I played in the barn with the chickens and their babies and watched the mice dart from here and there as the barn owl watched them from his perch high up in the rafters. The owl never moved while I was in the barn and must have hated me being in there messing with his hunting schedule. I was most happy there and felt the safest around the animals.

When another family showed up to visit with me one day, I did not understand why. Mrs. 'S.' awakened me early that morning and gave me a bath, then brushed out my hair. She told me these people were going to come and visit with me and that I was going to stay with them for a little while. I was also warned not to tell them any of my stupid little stories or they would know and I would be in really big trouble when I got home. I promised I wouldn't as she put me in an outfit I had never seen before. I was told to sit quietly and wait until they arrived and not to get dirty. I was allowed to sit on the sofa in the living room as I waited for the new people to arrive. They finally drove into the driveway in a big car and got out. I watched the man and the woman walk to the house and heard Mrs. 'S.' greet them with such a nice voice, it made me jump a little. They walked into the living room and looked at me for a moment. The lady walked over to me and knelt in front of me and held out her hand. She told me her name and asked me if I would like to come with them for a visit; to which I replied that I would like to. I followed them out to their car with Mrs. 'S.' calling after me to behave myself. I said that I would but I knew it really meant 'Keep your mouth shut!' They took me to their hotel for the first visit, which I assumed was their home and I was quite impressed! I went to a restaurant with them for dinner and was amazed at all the food there was. I don't remember much else from the visit except being grilled by the 'Smith's' when I got back and promising that I didn't tell the new people anything. I told my sister that I had told them all about her and she was happy and hugged me. She said something about them maybe being our new parents but I really didn't understand what she meant. When the people came for a second visit, I was quite ill and they visited me at the foster home where I lay on the sofa during the short visit. I remember the lady stroking my hair and that it felt nice as she spoke softly to me. They were never told I was sick due to Mr. and a few buddies deciding it would be funny to force-feed beer to me the night before. I had alcohol poisoning, but they were told I had the flu. In late November of 1970, Mrs. 'Smith' was sitting me on her lap for the first time ever and was being really nice to me while brushing my long, curly black hair. She was busily telling me how much she loved me, would miss me and that I was going to go to live with a new family who would love me too. I questioned whether my sister was coming too but was told that they didn't want my sister as she was 'bad', so I must remember to be a good girl, or they would not want me either. I remembered and believed those words for my entire childhood and was constantly afraid I'd be given up. My sister had been taken away while I was still asleep, so I never had a chance to say goodbye. I went up to our room with Mrs. 'Smith' and we packed what little I had in a tiny suitcase and I waited for the social worker to come. I later was informed that the 'Smith' family had over two hundred children placed with them over the years. I shudder to think how many they abused. I also became one of thousands of children involved in a multi – million-dollar law suit against the Ministry of Social Services, which will be years before it's settled. I have made it clear that I expect no settlement and am happy with just the acknowledgement that I was abused.

· · • ○ • · ·

I was not allowed to say goodbye to my sister as she had already been taken away before I left, which greatly affected us both later in life. I was always afraid of family suddenly disappearing, while she resented and later hated me for being adopted. Her life was spent in foster homes, juvenile detention and later prison, while I was loaded up in the back of my Social Workers car to a new and wonderful life. I was driven for what seemed like forever as I sat in the back seat and looked out the window. On the way to my new home, it was repeated to me yet again by my social worker that this was to be my forever home and that these new people were going to adopt me. It was also reinforced that I must be a good girl or else I would be returned to the 'Smith' family. I kept watching out the car window on the way to my new home and wished I could run into the forests and escape as we drove by.

After being in the car for many hours, we finally arrived at a large brown house, which was to be my new home. It had a long driveway that went up a little hill and the house seemed to stretch out forever. I had a new father, mother, brother and grandparents, all of whom were strangers to me. I was shown through the house and to my very own room. Quite frankly, everything after that is a blur and I don't remember much, except fear. My new mother and I unpacked my little suite case and she asked me where all my toys were. I held up my little doll that I clutched in my hand and she said she was lovely. I had only gotten her the day before so I didn't really know how to play with my dolly but I held on to her for dear life. My new mother commented on how little clothing I had and said we would need to go shopping for some new clothes.

My new father was a doctor and my new mother a social worker; this was to be very useful in the future. She would recognize behaviors in me which led her to questioning my background. She also had a better understanding than most how to handle me, and thank goodness, she did. My brother and I developed a relatively normal relationship, with typical sibling behaviors and rivalry. My grandfather was a serious man, who always seemed to be cross with someone or something, but

I adored him and I know it was reciprocated. My middle name was changed to that of my grandmothers' middle name and I liked that idea as well. I remember sitting in the judge's chambers and being asked if I liked my new name. I did and it was permanently changed, I became a legal member of the family.

I was not like other children who would laugh and play, run around and be children. I knew nothing of toys, play or how to be a little girl. My new father and Mother were gentle and kind and I simply did not understand this. I lived in constant terror of doing something wrong, so the first few months I did my best to be perfect. If I thought I had made a mistake over something, I would erupt into tears becoming inconsolable, thinking I was on my way back to the 'Smith' home.

In many respects, I believe I could have had a happy, normal, middle-class upbringing in that I had wonderful parents and a typical brother. Had I not been so severely damaged by the time they adopted me, I could have settled in nicely and moved on with my new life. We lived in a large house, had the freedom to play but the structure of music lessons and sports, friends and education. We pretty much had the idyllic life that one could easily compare to the 'Cosby Family'. My brother and I were blessed with hardworking parents who did their very best to provide everything we would need to become well-adjusted adults. There was church on Sundays, Sunday dinner with the grandparents, Friday night homemade pizza in front of the television and even a dog and a cat. From the outside, everything looked perfect and for the most part was, except for me. Every summer we would pack the family car and tow a trailer around the country side on vacations that where wonderful, yet educational as well. I must admit I was always a little surprised when they brought me back with them, half expecting to be left behind somewhere.

From all appearances, I presented as an average child. I was a pretty little girl with a great smile and a talent for music. Many people thought I sang like an angel and I enjoyed the adulation I received when I performed. I played the part of the little angel when with others and when I was required to do so at functions, church etc. Manipulation came very easy to me and I relished in the ability to make people do what I wanted just with a sweet smile. I remember people at church thinking what a little darling I was while I was thinking of ways they might die. It wouldn't necessarily involve my killing them, but sometimes natural deaths as well. Death was a recurrent theme for me, a means of permanent escape, although I didn't necessarily understand where we went when we died. I knew we went away from 'here'. It seemed to me like it could be wonderful there and I might be happier there. It was also a place I could send people who annoyed me or that I disliked. I never told anyone this, but death was never far from my thoughts. It was because of these thoughts that later on in life I worried that I might be capable of murder or be a Psychopath, but with years of learning I have come to understand that I am neither. While I agree that these are not normal thoughts for a young child, considering my past history, it was not farfetched, nor was I normal!

I was happiest when I was alone. Children my own age didn't understand me nor I them, as they had never had to fight to survive like I had. I had difficulty understanding games and remembering rules, so that left me in the cold when they played. Unfortunately, I was also far advanced in some experiences no child should be. So, when they played as children, it was foreign to me and childish. While their dolls were babies and they were the mommies, my dolls were having sexual intercourse and oral sex in random encounters in my Barbie camper. I never really knew how to play mommy, but I knew how to play wife or girlfriend. When my mother noticed I did not play with my dolls normally and often found them naked in adult positions, she began to question more about my history. When she questioned the Children's Aide in the community from where I had come, they denied any knowledge and suggested she was making things up or didn't know what she was talking about. They even told her to send me back if she was unhappy, like I was some replaceable toy. It wasn't until years later that I finally opened up and told her much of the truth. For many years following my adoption, I never said a word, as I feared being beaten, taken back or given away. Even though my family never abused me, it was always in the back of my mind that I could be or even worse; I could be returned to the 'Smith's'.

This is where the additional diagnosis of Post-Traumatic Stress Disorder came from, understandably. I wasn't diagnosed with this until much later, after I divulged the sexual and physical abuse to a psychiatrist. He likened it to the equivalent of a war survivor who had undergone torture and, in a sense, I had. I just didn't experience the war. I still wake up at night occasionally with night sweats and terrors.

My imagination was immense and safe. I could take myself anywhere and actually be there in my mind. I could talk to the dog and the cat and understood them better than any person. I would fantasize about many other lives I might have and be content. Fantasy life was so very much easier than real life, as no one had any issues with me or me with them and I was completely accepted for who I was. I found it extremely difficult to pretend I was normal and trying to be like everyone else was next to impossible. When participating in family events, I would try to be the little princess, all perfect and behaved, but there was this other side to me that became excited - almost euphoric with the thought of burning down the world. I remember one day driving in the car with my dad and thinking I could stop the frustration of everything at school if I just got out of the car. I unbuckled my seatbelt and opened the door preparing to just get out…of a moving vehicle. My father had to slam on the breaks, reached across me and shut my door. He yelled "What the hell are you doing?" my response? "I don't know". How could I explain I needed everything to stop? I mean everything, my entire world, because I was stuck and lost. My father kept the car doors locked after that episode, for fear I might try again.

When in the car driving along the highway, I loved to look at the trees and forested areas we would pass. I would imagine running away from home and hiding in the forest, living off the land under a make-shift shelter of twigs and branches. I was aware enough that there would not be the conveniences that I had experienced with this family, however that never bothered me. I had lived off garbage before when at my last foster home as we were always starving. I was always very sure of my own survival and never gave it a second thought.

When my parents would scold me for misbehaving, I actually was glad when they sent me to my room, as then I would be left alone to my own imagination. The funny thing was in my imagination I was alone there too, except for the animals. In my imagination and in real life, I had incredible relationships with animals. I knew I was safe with them and they seemed to sense something in me. I was able to engage a neighbor's dog that was usually unfriendly with everyone else. While they were chased away, I was giving her belly rubs. I was never afraid with animals and felt far safer with them than people. If bitten by a dog, I was never angry with it but felt sorry for making it frightened of me, this would lead to my feelings of despair knowing I had caused fear in the animal. I can't explain why it mattered so much to me that I might hurt an animal yet caused excitement in me at the thought of hurting people. I can only say that people had already hurt me so badly yet, animals never had. People in my eyes deserved to be hurt, mutilated and destroyed, but animals did not. At a young age, I understood that people lied, manipulated, hurt, destroyed each other. They had done so much damage to me that I hated people and to an extent still do. It has affected my ability to trust, form friendships and relationships as well and honestly, no wonder! I must admit that part of my distaste for people also comes from my inability at times to understand them or read their facial expressions. They can be very confusing to me and contradict what the person is saying. As well, being hearing impaired, I don't always hear what they are saying. It's amazing to me how many people also talk while covering or masking their mouths. This makes lip reading impossible. When you add facial expressions not matching what they are saying, I often wonder how much I am really misunderstanding. If I think they are being sarcastic or mean, I will smile and walk away. I have been mistaken a few times and had people think me rude, but I am ok with that and correct it later. I am not comfortable being forced to endure an unpleasant scene and will always walk away. This had led me to become more self-aware and protective, finally.

The ability to recognize dangerous situations or people is extremely worrisome for parents and this is a definite side effect of FASD. We really don't understand danger and have an almost fatalistic sense of immortality. If we are told not to do something because it's dangerous or we might get hurt, it becomes a challenge to accomplish it. We can play with matches because we won't get burned. We can talk to strangers, no one wants to abduct us because no one wants us. We can climb higher in the tree because we won't fall. It is far better to take away the harm than to expect us to stay away from it. Lock away lighters and matches, cut the low hanging limbs from the tree and hold our hands in public. You may also consider putting locks on windows and doors so they only open so far, keep harmful chemicals behind locked doors and all medications out of our reach. This is most important during our teenage years as well, please don't think we will know any better then either! We might know better but the challenge will still be there and our brains don't have that switch!

I had difficulty understanding limitations and never did understand the 'no talking to strangers' rule. I would take risks, climb the highest trees and was quite the tomboy. I can't say I had no sense of my own mortality because I knew what death was, I was just never afraid of it. I am still not afraid of death and often look forward to it. Am I suicidal now? Absolutely not, I love my children too much to be that selfish. I am just not afraid of this life ending. By the same token, I am not fatalistic either. I still plan for my future, have goals to accomplish and life to live. I also have beliefs about what comes next and have found great comfort in my unusual faith. I can say I have been able to find honesty and peace in my faith, where others have left me questioning and empty. I have also found love, healing and a real sense of belonging; isn't that what faith is supposed to be about?

When I was six years old my brother and I were playing outside together. I was running down the big hill in the front yard while I was laughing; I tripped over my feet and fell very hard. I did not cry or tell my parents until that evening when the pain became too much and my shoulder began to swell. My mother had come in to say goodnight to me and I had begun to cry in pain after she touched me. So off we went to the doctor's office and had X-rays done in the late evening. I had a badly broken collar bone and they were amazed I had not spoken out earlier. This was also one of the many indicators that something was quite different about me. I was stuck wearing my brother's t-shirts, as nothing else would fit over my butterfly sling to stabilize my collar bone. My poor mother had just finished sewing quite a few little sun dresses for me and I couldn't wear any of them. By the time I was healed, not one of the dresses fit me anymore. The point to this is that my pain threshold was and still is to the extreme. When one has experienced physical abuse, one learns to shut certain feelings off and sometimes, emotions as well. They are the toughest to find again, if we ever can.

When I became frightened or overly anxious about something, I would develop a high fever and become nauseated. I was nauseous every morning at breakfast and much to my brother's dismay would often result in my breakfast reappearing all over the table and myself.

At times, it could be difficult to tell if I was upset about something or had the flu, but somehow my parents figured it out.

My parents held Christmas dessert parties every year before the 25th, for neighbors, associates and friends. My mother would be busily baking for days prior, while we decorated the house and cleaned up. There would be cookies, cakes, pies, puddings and candies everywhere amidst the decorations and people laughing and chatting. My first party I spent hiding as much as I could, but in later years dressed in matching mother-daughter outfits, learning to play the little hostess.

· · · ○ · · ·

Christmas has gone from being one of my worst and most traumatic memories to my best. My first Christmas was challenging, confusing and startling. I quietly watched as the real tree was put in place and decorated with all the trimmings. I saw many colorfully wrapped presents placed in great piles under the tree and I was filled with dread. Christmas was not a happy time for me but one of terror instead. I didn't know what would happen in this new place but I was sure I wasn't going to be happy. I came out of my room in the morning after being awakened by my brother and went to the dimly lit living room. The Christmas tree was lit with blinking bulbs and tinsel sparkling everywhere, it was so pretty. The presents were piled higher than I had ever seen and we had stockings that were so heavy and overflowing that they were laid in the big chairs next to the fireplace. It looked better than a department store Christmas display or any television commercial ever! My brother dug into his stocking and I watched as he ate some candy and ripped through his stocking. He motioned for me to do the same thing but I was terrified I would be punished. Finally, I found a Barbie doll lying amongst the overflow of my stocking. I removed her from her box and sat in the chair with her until my parents got up. My mother explained to me that I could go through everything in the stocking, as it was all for me. I was sure it was a trick or they would yell at me for touching it, it was beyond my imagination. Inside I found trinkets, candy, an enormous orange and the biggest red delicious apple that I had ever seen, more trinkets, candy and tinker toys. I was over whelmed and quite happy eating the candies before they could be taken away, or so I thought. I inhaled as much of the apple as I could, it was just as sweet as all that candy! We were told we must wait for Grandma and Grandpa to arrive before we could open presents, but I was so busy with my new Barbie and other trinkets I didn't really hear or understand.

When they finally arrived, and settled in, I remember crying at one point because my mother kept trying to get me to set Barbie down and open more wonderful presents. I couldn't understand that all those presents under the tree were for me! I was simply overwhelmed. I received a shiny red and white tricycle which I quickly learned to ride and absolutely loved for years! My mother had spent hours looking for a brown haired, brown eyed doll just like me and I hardly noticed her. I opened packages with beautiful dresses and outfits that would fill my closet, games, books and yet more toys. I truly don't remember any other gifts than the ones I've mentioned, although I know there was so much more. After opening everything my mother asked me what my favorite gift was and I replied that I loved my Barbie and would be happy with that. I also informed her that I would pack up everything else to be given away as I knew I wouldn't be allowed to keep it all. To my amazement she told me I would be keeping it all and that I was allowed to play with all of it. I think it took a few months before I really played with it all!

I remember my first Christmas dinner as my favorite part of the day. I initially sat at the kitchen table and quietly waited while all the food was set out. I just assumed I wouldn't be allowed to sit at the pretty table in the dining room and expected to sit in the kitchen for my meal. Finally, when all was set, my father came into the kitchen and asked me if I was coming to the table and I followed him into the dining room, amazed I was allowed to sit at the table with everyone else. It was beautiful with all its glittering crystal, silver, china, candles and so much food. I ate turkey, mashed potatoes, vegetables I had never seen before and even a casserole with marshmallows on top! Then came dessert, which was a pudding with carrots in it smothered in a delicious vanilla sauce…I was in heaven! I was exhausted at the end of the day and I believe perhaps suffering from a food coma. I am sure you understand when I tell you my mother was an absolutely amazing cook and worked magic with Christmas dinners. I don't ever remember a bad Christmas except when the dog tried to eat the ham one year.

I now make myself too busy to remember Christmas past and I have the dessert parties at our home. I now cook the Christmas dinner with the sparkling crystal, silver, china and candles. For the most part I hope and believe no one has any idea the torture and triumph I wrestle with every year. Although I still find it extremely stressful, I love the decorations and ceremony of family Christmas. I endeavor each year to carry on the traditions I have been given.

If I can give advice here, if you adopt an older child, take it easy the first Christmas and birthday. Try not to overwhelm them with every possible gift in the world and take it slowly. Watch how they are handling the day and if they need a break, let them have it, everything will still be there! You might also wish to limit the people during the first day of the holidays, and maybe spread get togethers out over a few days. It's easy to lose track of a new child amongst large families and you want to check in with your new addition and see they are ok. Sometimes they might not want to leave your side, then please let them cling. Everything is so very new and they need to know you are the one constant that will not change. At the same time, it is important to limit their alone time as you need to let them know you have not forgotten them. They will test you on this most certainly!

Each child is going to be different, yet have the same need to please and fit in, while feeling safe. This last point may take some time and you will need to know as much history as possible for the child. As painful as it may be to hear, you need to know if your child had been sexually interfered with or abused. They will be looking at you with the same eyes as they looked at their abusers with and you will be under scrutiny. They will expect you to hurt them and be confused with you if you don't. Remember, this is what they know and they need to learn a different way of life that does not include pain. This is where counselling for the whole family can be so very valuable. It can teach you how to cope with the pain your child has suffered and be supportive yet place limits on expectations for all of you.

Bath time can also be so difficult for new parents when their child has been sexually abused. One of the first things my mother taught me was to wash myself and that no one needed to help me. I was quite capable of washing between my legs myself and that no one had the right to do so but me! She would help me with my hair, back, elbows and knees, but I could do the rest. I could dry myself and put on my pajamas myself as well, then climb into bed with the covers pulled up, to await my story. I taught my children the exact same way she taught me.

What is a Meltdown?

───────── • • • ○ • • • ─────────

LITTLE BILLY IS IN THE checkout line with Mommy screaming something inaudible when he throws himself on the floor and proceeds to scream and cry uncontrollably. Others in the line start suggesting that this spoiled brat needs a good spanking or more! Of course, this is the furthest thing from the truth, little Billy is having a meltdown! So, what is a meltdown anyways and what are the causes that make FASD kids explode into irrational little, uncontrollable, screaming monsters? When trying to come up with a simplistic answer I quickly realized it was not possible. Outwardly, it is a child kicking and screaming, uncontrolled in a rage of tears, who is inconsolable by words or actions of the parents, caregivers or teachers. They are as result often forcibly restrained or locked in a room so they can't hurt themselves or others. It's when uninformed adults say 'That child needs a good kick in the ass!' or 'a good spanking!' Trying to explain to a normal, average individual what is happening inside one's brain and body during this chaos is like trying to explain a war scene in a movie with hundreds of actors, giving each individual actor's point of view at the exact same time. It is a series of things which culminate into a full blown, uncontrolled meltdown and I will try to list <u>some</u> of them here.

Firstly, it is about us being over stimulated and experiencing muscle aches with no way to release it. My Dad, the Doctor, thought it might be a combination of a buildup of Nitric Oxide and dehydration in the muscle tissue. Sometimes it's similar to a Charlie horse- only not quite as severe, just nagging. Other times it can be agonizing pain that will not stop. It can be over the entire body, just in the legs, or sometimes just in the face (yes literally) which is why you see us opening our mouths wide like a snake preparing to struggle down a meal twice its size. We also can be seen making faces, scrunching our eyes tightly and clenching our jaws. It feels like you are about to run a race and your muscles are preparing to go the distance. You know you need to get rid of the ache, but don't know how or aren't allowed to. Sometimes this muscle ache is accompanied by chills along the spine as well as the sense of needing to repeat one certain physical behavior numerous times. This is where I use meditation techniques, now that I am more aware of what is happening, to relieve the aches. I often recommend Yoga or running to release the chemicals in the rest of the muscles.

Secondly, it's the amygdala in the brain not doing its job because it's damaged. The amygdala according to Science Daily is "an almond-shape set of neurons located deep in the brain's medial temporal lobe. Shown to play a key role in the processing of emotions, the amygdala forms part of the limbic system. In humans and other animals, this subcortical brain structure is linked to both fear responses and pleasure...Its size is positively correlated with aggressive behavior across species. Conditions such as anxiety, autism, depression, post-traumatic stress disorder, and phobias are suspected of being linked to abnormal functioning of the amygdala, owing to damage, developmental problems, or neurotransmitter imbalance (1)." So now that you have the scientific version, let me put it in FASD language – it's damaged and therefore we CAN'T regulate emotions properly. Understand the word <u>can't</u> here, it is not a choice; our little flippy flopper is damaged and <u>does not work</u> properly! It is broken and can never be repaired!

This part is most frustrating for others as people have a need to 'fix' things and other people. When faced with a problem that has no simple solution, people become frustrated and tend to give up. When something is irrevocably broken, we tend to buy new, but when it can't be purchased what then? No one should live with something that's broken, so let's find a way to fix it. It's a vicious cycle. Until people accept it for what it is; brain damage, they will never move on to what's really important which is how to DEAL with it.

Thirdly, it's frustration because we can't understand you or be understood by you. It's about concepts or math problems that are Greek to us after the fifteenth explanation. It's also about the teacher who is giving the fifteenth explanation and is frustrated we don't understand a simplistic math equation. It's about expectations that are far too high for us to achieve in the time frame you or others expect. It's about feeling things we don't understand or not feeling things we're supposed to. It's about knowing you will never measure up or achieve what your parents hope for. It's about wars in the world and the world ending. It's about us dying and yet not understanding death. It's about whether we're going to heaven or hell when we die. It's about our parents fighting and are they going to divorce or the pain of divorce and wanting to be with both parents. It's about competing with the perfect sibling we have or another child in the classroom or being compared to them. It's about a sound that is painful or a touch or lights that hurt. It's about dreams at night that would scare the hell out of any adult, but we get to experience them as children. It's about memories or experiences we can't share because of fear. It's the fear of being rejected and knowing we must reject you first, that way it won't hurt as much. It's about not being able to make friends or not understanding why they are no longer your friends. It's being terrified of the bully at school or terrified because you are the bully and don't know why, not to mention can't stop. It's also about not being able to turn off the world and it going 90 miles an hour without us. We are thinking all this at the same time plus more except it's a jumbled mess that we can't begin to sort out because we don't know where the beginning is or the end.

Lastly, it is the total lack of control of our lives. Everyone is telling us what is wrong with us, what we are doing wrong, how we're doing it wrong, how we are thinking wrong, how we need to improve, how we need to correct and what we must do next. None of which we can begin to understand. Someone is constantly hanging on to us with an iron grip or we're stuck wearing a harness or we have parents or teachers yelling at us to stay close or back up a bit, we are too close. People ask us why and we don't know why but they expect us to have all the answers and get frustrated when we say 'I don't know'. 'What do you mean you don't know- you did it?' Well folks, we really don't know why except to say our brains said to do it and we COULD NOT resist it or our brains said to stop and we COULD NOT. To expect us to tell you why is unreasonable because we don't know why our brains are misfiring. The amount of negative we hear far surpasses any positive feedback even in our own minds, as we tell ourselves we're useless, stupid or retarded. If you're an adult saying anything negative it multiplies exponentially in our brain to infinity and beyond!

Now mix all this together at once and you have a meltdown. The result of all this is a flight or fight response that <u>must</u> be acted upon, we do not have any choice in this. It literally feels like we are drowning or dying if we don't. There is no freeze response or wait, it is immediate and uncontrollable. There is no off button to shut it down - it must be played out to relieve the pain, to the point of exhaustion. Yes, it is painful and yes, it is exhausting for us and no, we have no control over it any more than an epileptic seizure. I am exhausted after just writing this part alone because of the familiarity of it.

When the meltdown is over, many parents are still fired up and now they want answers as to why that just happened. This will serve nothing except to fire us up again, so don't do it! We need to have a chance to recover and sleep. It really is much like a seizure in that you would not ask an epileptic to run a marathon after a seizure, so why would you try to enter into a thoughtful discussion with someone who is both mentally and physically exhausted. Give us time to recover, like a few days and then carefully, gently approach.

There is a way to prevent the meltdown which is recognizing the symptoms at the onset, asking <u>simple</u> questions like "are you achy?" or "does your neck feel funny?" Watch for signs like twitching or fidgeting, frustration or being argumentative. You will see their discomfort and although they might not be capable of verbalizing it so it's up to you to suggest physical distractions that they enjoy. Stop doing what you are doing and change gears, distract! Give the child the opportunity to do yoga or running or some other physical activity to clear the chemical build up in the muscles, which can also help distract or clear the mind. You might also try rhythmic drumming as it gets the child to focus on a rhythm and helps focus the mind better. You must ask if the child feels achy, frustrated or needs a time out or a run period. You must also be able to allow the child to complete this and not simply put the child in a room so they don't hurt themselves or others, which is what many schools are doing.

You know what you would like us to accomplish, so give us options and choices instead of telling us. If we need to complete Math, English and Spelling, ask us which we would like to do first. Does it really matter if Math is completed by 9:20 a.m.? If you want us to clean our rooms, ask us to pick up the white socks only and place them in the red basket then tell us to pick up the blacks socks and put them in the blue basket, but please do not tell us to just clean our rooms as it's too overwhelming. Do not give us lists any longer than three items or we will forget. Three is our limit and on a bad day we can't even handle three!

Repetition and routine are our friends and we thrive on them. It's ok to set our lives to a schedule but give us many opportunities to choose. Would you like purple socks today or pink ones, that's a fabulous choice, well done! Praise us for the little things we do accomplish as for us they might be huge! Half an hour of any subject we struggle with is fifteen minutes too long, let us have fifteen minutes then a little five- or ten-minute break before we have to regroup and try again. Think outside the box and be inventive, we have to just to get through the next five minutes and some days it's everything we can do to accomplish that!

The funny thing is when I explained my meltdown description to my Autistic son; he agreed immediately that I had nailed it on the head. I hadn't realized in the writing of my own FASD description, I was describing what an Autistic meltdown was like as well. After all, both diagnoses are under the Pervasive Development Disorder umbrella, so it would make sense there would also be similarities in symptoms. If I tried to explain to you just how difficult this chapter was to write, I would have to explain that it took me a few months just to isolate each component of the meltdown in order to identify it and I didn't add every thought in our heads as that would have been a book in itself!. I now need to tackle something simpler before I can continue writing…maybe I'll clean my room.

The bottom line is that as one ages, we learn coping skills so the meltdowns come less and less over time. Of course, we still struggle but as well as growing older we are given more responsibility and therefore able to make more choices, which in the end is what we are fighting for. It's ok for your child to fail and learn from a mistake as this is how they retrain their damaged brain. Keeping the mistakes simple and not harmful is obviously imperative, but we have to be able to choose to screw up. We have made some interesting things around here through making mistakes. When working with kids and their dogs I give the children three options for correcting the dog's behavior, one option is the correct answer, one option is incorrect and the third option is just plain nonsense. The child is aware I'm being silly, but they still show great pride in choosing for themselves. So, what if it is obvious- let them have it, it's good for the ego. I have also given them options for their own behavior by telling them if you're angry, you can yell, hit a punching bag or kick a ball and they choose. Some days they come and don't feel like working with their dog, so they get the options of building a birdhouse, making some pudding or working with the dog. I have quite a few birdhouses, worked with many dogs and then enjoyed some delicious pudding with the kids. What a fun day and we accomplished everything on the list. We also accomplished reading, mathematics and spelling on the side!

We also never end a session with a child and their dog on a bad note. Every session is ended with them receiving encouragement, praise and giving their dog treats, play and belly rubs. It encourages pride in the child for a job well done, as well as the bond to develop between the child and the dog; everyone goes home looking forward to the next visit here. We have many parents tell us that Jr. couldn't wait to get here today and was talking all the way here about what they might do today. Inevitably they learn something new every time they come and enjoy the learning as well.

I will state irrefutably that educators need to be educated on teaching techniques for children with F.A.S.D. So often I appear before principals, teachers and educational assistants who, through lack of information, are attempting to teach and manage behaviors of children with F.A.S.D. like they would any other child. Often, they equate Autism and F.A.S.D. as one in the same behaviorally and this could not be farther from the truth! This simply does not work and they arc left with frustrated, angry children who rebel or simply get lost in the system.

For those who do not understand the difference between these two diagnoses, let me explain it simply. Most FASD children have a behavioral switch that gets stuck in the 'on' position and they can't turn it off. They know it's there; they know it's stuck and they know their behavior is wrong but they cannot stop it. Autistic children have no idea there is even a switch in the first place.

There are many educated and informed professionals in both Canada and the United States who are ready and willing to share proven methodology for teaching children with F.A.S.D. However, until Educational Boards accept the fact that there are many children falling through the cracks because of misinformation or worse, ignorance or denial of the problem existing, I am afraid many more children will be harmed. And they are being harmed!

This wording may seem as excessive to some, however when police are routinely called to a school because a child has become so frustrated, they become physically violent with staff, the word 'excessive' no longer applies. So often this frustration can be avoided by utilizing proven, demonstrated techniques and thus the violence need never occur. I often use many of these methods when working with children and find myself wishing they had been present when I attended school. Perhaps school would have been a more pleasant experience for me than the torture it really was.

School Daze

— • • ● ○ ● • • —

As it was, I began school shortly after being adopted by my family at age five. I attended kindergarten like every other child and enjoyed my first year in school. From there my educational experience quickly went downhill and never really recovered. In grade one, I was unfortunate enough to be given a teacher who soon 'diagnosed' me as retarded and told me thus. She regularly chastised me in front of the class, leaving me in tears at my desk. She seemed to delight in my misery and I very quickly began to hate going to school. She would keep me after school berating me as to how stupid and retarded, I was, until my mother caught her in the act one day. My mother rescued me and dealt with the situation by speaking to the Principle, however after that day the teacher basically ignored me altogether.

My mother was back then, and still is, a wonderfully formidable woman who could make any school administrator shake in their boots. My brother and I used to refer to her as 'putting her war bonnet on' and were just relieved not to be on the receiving end! As children we knew that it was great to have a mom who could almost make the principle cry, or so we thought!

I had few friends in the first grade and seemed to gravitate towards the 'strange' kids. My sixth birthday party was made up of a collection of 'Oliver Twist's, Huckleberry Finn's' and a few well placed 'Artful Dodger's'. I was able to pick out every abused, adopted, or neglected child in my class and invite them over for cake. My parents never said no to their attendance, but would quietly wince, and batten the hatches.

I never received any testing in school for learning disorders so was not diagnosed until I was in my twenties. Instead, it was assumed I was lazy, uncooperative or just plain disinterested. My elementary years were consumed with extreme bouts of anxiety and frustration that often led to me running away from school during lunch or afternoon recess. I would run home and sneak into the house where, inevitably, our housekeeper would find me and share some cookies with me. I never got in trouble for running away and this may actually be new information for my parents when they read this book. I did not do it often, but admit to it occurring at least once per month. One day my third-grade teacher observed me heading for the hills and sent a large group of children in hot pursuit which absolutely terrified me. I spent the rest of the day sitting in the cloakroom shaking until it was time to go home.

I did not make many friends although I did have one throughout elementary school. Janice and I were best friends and enjoyed sleepovers like other kids. Through Janice, I learned how to play with dolls and games for the first time in my life. She would sometimes help me with my school work and became my best friend for a few years. For the most part however, I was somewhat of a loner throughout my school years and did not really relate well to the children my own age. Although I had periods of loneliness and often wished for a friend, I also never pursued one as I knew they would not last, as my ability to trust would result in me sabotaging the friendship.

I did excel at school in English, art, music and history, as I loved these subjects and would spend hours on them. Math was my arch nemesis and I hopelessly, repeatedly failed at it. For me it was like trying to learn a second language and I was constantly struggling. My father would try to help me which usually ended with me in tears of frustration. It would not matter how many times he explained a process, I simply could not grasp it. We now know that I have learning disabilities which affected my organizational skills, math skills and short-term memory loss, but at the time it was an unknown. I have since learned to approach math differently and have become quite adept at doing simple math in my head. I was fortunate in grade eight to have a teacher who paired my musical talent with learning mathematics. He had me writing songs for math equations and I received an 80% in math that year. He was my only favorite teacher and was quite an advocate for me with the other teachers. I still contact him occasionally to this day!

In high school, I maintained good grades in English, geography, history, music and art, while math and sciences fell apart. After falling behind and mounting behavioral issues, in grade eleven my parents sent me to a Theatre Arts School in Toronto, where I could concentrate on music and theatre. It was an entirely new world of freedom and I took full advantage of being in Toronto but it was not in favor of my school work. Eventually the school itself crumbled due to mismanagement and I was sent back home. I spent about a month and a half at home before I ran away back to Toronto. I had to finish my diploma later in my twenties.

Suffice to say in all my years in school, I had only the one teacher who recognized the need to teach outside the parameters of the proverbial box and try different techniques to help me. I often wonder why there was only one who had the imagination or desire to do so.

I also had a guitar teacher who was my biggest supporter musically. I adored 'Tony' and he always made me feel as though it was mutual. I remember him teaching me a song from Holland that his mother used to sing to him in Dutch. While I had no idea what I was singing, I know I made him cry every time I sang it. Tony often had me performing during sidewalk sale days in our home town in front of his store. He always said I was worth thousands in advertising! He was always so gentle with me and greeted me with a huge smile. He often called me his little peacock because when I sang it was like watching me spread my feathers. I adored my father, my grandfather, Tony and Mr. Robar, my favorite teacher. They were amongst the first men in my life who just liked me for me, nothing more and they just saw the potential in me.

I was an avid reader as a child and thoroughly enjoyed the escape books offered me. I could read for hours and daydream even longer. I could closely relate to Anne of Green Gables and solve crimes with the Hardy Boys. My imagination kept me engaged and became a substitute when reality became overwhelming. I was and still am an avid writer and was frequently given high marks for my stories. In art class, I developed talent in drawing skills and have subsequently sold a few pieces. Many of us diagnosed with F.A.S.D. have artistic skills and show talent with music or other abilities. I was fortunate to have parents who recognized my musical abilities and provided piano, guitar and voice lessons. Through music I learned that I could be good at something and this gave my self-confidence an essential boost. I earned many awards and scholarships at music festivals and enjoyed learning to play other instruments and playing in bands. I did not pursue a career in music much to my parents' disappointment; however, I still enjoy it.

• • • ○ • • •

In terms of the personal side of my life during this time, I felt as though I was still trying to fit within the mold my foster parents suggested in order to remain with my new family. The idea that my new family loved me and wouldn't send me packing still lived with me daily and I was constantly trying to prove myself unlovable. I spent the first few years hiding my physical pains from falls and normal injuries, as any child sustains in daily life. I could not be a weak child as that was simply unacceptable as far as I believed. I tried to do my best at everything but admittedly hated organized physical activity and gym class at school. Structured games with rules did not sit well with me and I truly hated them. I excelled at the loner sports, and became quite a good swimmer. The phrase 'Does not play well with others' certainly applied to me and I was the first to admit it! I also hated physical contact in my early years and did everything to avoid it. I remember trying to squirm out of hugs from my parents as I really did not understand what they meant, nor did I enjoy them. When I was over stimulated, they became painful, as though my skin were on fire. I remember one time actually taking sandpaper from my Dad's workbench and rubbing it on my arms hoping to make the burn go away and I found that the sting of the scraped skin was actually a preferable sensation to the burn. I had great difficulty in distinguishing sensations as well and found that I preferred pain over all. I truly 'felt' pain instead of wishy-washy feelings of emotions. At times my muscles still felt achy for no reason, or at least I couldn't figure out why. It wasn't until I attended diving camp where I learned about self-relaxation techniques and meditation, that I found relief.

I was taught by my instructor how to tighten, hold and relax muscle groupings ascending from my feet all the way to my head, in a rhythmic method. For the first time in my life, I found relief for those damnable aches I felt all my life when I was over stimulated or anxious. The aching sensations often led me to hurt myself or others, as I was trying to accomplish the same thing as taught to me through meditation. I see this so often in other children with F.A.S.D. and recommend Yoga to their parents as quickly as I can! Many parents want to place their children in Karate or some other martial art and my response is 'Why teach them how to hurt others better?' Yoga is a wonderful series of non-violent exercises in self relaxation, awareness and also teaches control. It has taught me a lot about breathing techniques, muscle isolation and relaxation; so that I have been able to live the life I have now. While I still get those aches, I now know how to relieve them safely without involving others or harming myself.

"Mom, I think she's dead" My mother heard my brother say as he burst into the house one wintery morning. Apparently, I had gone down our steep front hill on our toboggan and crashed face-first into a tree, knocking myself unconscious and chipping one of my teeth. Of course, I don't remember this having been unconscious, but I survived the experience nonetheless. I must explain that our front hill was fantastic for tobogganing, as one could race down it and then, if you steered the toboggan just so, you could catch air going up and over our driveway. It was marvelous and always felt like we were flying, although I tended to miss the driveway and always headed for that damnable tree. I was sure at times, the tree intentionally stepped *into* my path, despite my brother repeatedly teaching me to steer the toboggan. The tree also ruthlessly aimed for me when I was learning to ride my bicycle, as my brother positioned me at the top of the hill and pushed. He never told me I had to steer that too. Despite the mishaps with the tree, I learned to climb it better than my brother and decided it was better to be in the tree, than the tree wearing me.

In behind our house was a lush green pasture for the neighbor's cattle that seemed to go on forever, and I loved to go walking through it, rain or shine. I adored the cow's soft velvety muzzles and gentle nature I had learned about at the 'Smith's'. I never forgot my cow friend I had made at my last foster home and made quite a few friends in our neighbor's herd as well. At the back of the pasture stood a small forest I loved to wander through and could easily be gone for hours. I always had a dog with me when I went on my adventures and learned very quickly that I could tell the dog anything. The dog was my best friend for a long time as well as the neighbors' dogs. They had a male and female pair named Nip and Tip, who inevitably had two litters of puppies. I would spend hours in the dog pen with momma and the pups, and come home filthy, but my mom would rarely complain about the dirty clothes.

I understood animals and could easily watch them for hours, imagining knowing exactly how they felt. They weren't complicated like people; they didn't care how you behaved or what the neighbors thought of you. They were simplistic, easy to please and I much preferred them to people. They also gave you warning if they were going to hurt you, so you had time to back off and give them space. Even the wild animals were simple and let me be relatively close. I never tried to touch them, except for the rabbits as I understood they were wild and would give a painful reminder if I got too close. I often fantasized about living in the woods in a makeshift hut and being with nature and the animals. If I wouldn't have missed candy bars so much, I might have wound up doing so, but alas, chocolate won and pizza and cookies and…

I also learned about new foods, and found out about muffins, ice-cream sundaes (it's not gravy on top, but actually chocolate sauce!) and learned to love my father's oatmeal. I still occasionally became ill at breakfast, much to my parent's dismay and my brother's gross-out limit, but eventually I managed it. I learned about my dad's stew and that it is was the best in the world, homemade pizza on Friday nights, the bakery's warm donuts on Saturday mornings and going for lunch after church on Sunday. My dad almost always had liver and onions, at which we all groaned and wrinkled our noses.

I rarely cried from the pain of hurting myself in typical childhood mishaps or otherwise, and preferred to be alone. I did have a temper and was most stubborn. I could lose my temper, become frustrated and then uncontrollably enraged which resulted in lashing out at my mother. I know I hurt her physically a few times but I don't much remember these episodes very well. Apparently, I could become quite violent and on occasion required restraint so I would not hurt myself. Again, my knowledge of this is incomplete, as I would somehow detach myself from my surroundings during these episodes. I do know that at times during the beginning of these episodes, I could feel rather excited, almost high and powerful. It was impossible to stop at this point even though I knew I was wrong or should stop. My brain knew it but the message did not make it to the rest of my body, as though the wires connecting my brain with my behavior were cut. After the meltdowns, I would be exhausted and could not remember much of the tantrum. My mom and I would talk about it later and I would often agree that it didn't make any sense that I shouldn't have continued on in my rant but that I simply couldn't stop it. Even in the beginning of these tantrums I often knew I was wrong, but still could not end them before the situation became shear madness. This in itself frustrated me and left me feeling frenzied. Because of this I groped for anything I could control and clung to it ferociously. I could have days or even weeks of doing well and then suddenly would descend into madness, losing myself into the vicious cycle of irrationality all over again. I often wondered if I was 'crazy', but Mom explained this did not actually exist and was an inappropriate term. Luckily, she never gave me the appropriate term or I am sure I would have determined I was that. What I was in fact was an unhappy, undiagnosed kid who was barely understood by anyone including myself.

I was the worlds' best daydreamer, sometimes wandering astray for hours in my thoughts. In my dreams, I was someone else entirely and I was always happy. I was the pretty, popular girl with all the friends, the girl the boys all wanted to date, the girl the parents all admired, the perfect swimmer, singer, guitarist. I am sure most kids have dreams like this but reality inevitably came 'round and reminded me of who I really was. I never did feel comfortable in my skin and still don't. Sometimes it feels so wrong that my skin physically hurts and burns at someone's touch. This happens when I'm over stimulated, anxious or upset. My skin literally feels as though it's crawling and it hurts. My skin is normally hypersensitive and I am allergic to many things resulting in rashes or dry skin. If I become stressed, my left hand will dry out, crack and bleed. This was the hand that had been placed in some kind of boiling liquid when I was an infant or so the doctor thinks. I have scarring on my hand which is most visible during the summer when I am tanned.

The abuse I experienced in the foster home inevitably led to sexual dysfunction and definite promiscuity as I grew older, as well as significant confusion with regards to sex verses love. I could not understand why my adoptive parents did not repeat this abuse with me. For me, violence, sexual abuse and love were all the same thing. One could not exist without the others. As result, for years I did not believe my parents really loved me and when I was older, I sought out these types of relationships. It was difficult for me to understand relationships and I destroyed many of them along the way, as well as picking inappropriate partners, when I eventually became sexually active. I looked for what I knew, violence and abuse and I found far too many partners willing to fulfil this expectation. This lack of understanding became a major factor in leading to unhealthy relationships, rape and abusive relationships. I have experienced true rape a few times in my life and discovered when it happened in my older years, I simply detached myself from my body and went on afterward like it was just another normal day. I don't really know that it affected me emotionally as it had become such a normal part of life when I was a child prior to being adopted, so it only seemed natural to me as an adult. The disgust and disbelief I are sure you are experiencing with this statement might be overwhelming for you and I apologize, but for me this statement just…is.

· · · ○ · · ·

I was overly friendly with strangers and almost got myself into dangerous situations because of this. My mother worked with many of the police officers in town because of her job as a social worker. One day she received a call from them. I was walking home from school and saw a man feeding squirrels in the park. I went over to talk to him and he seemed nervous, asking me to go away. When I got home my Mom spoke to me about the incident saying that I had been seen talking to a known pedophile in the park, and they had let him know they were watching him so he would send me off on my way without harm. I believe I wrecked their case that day, and my mothers' nerves. Another time I was down by the road in front of our house talking to strangers in a car, when my dad yelled and they sped off. My mother was sure it was my biological maternal donor attempting to do goodness knows what. Suffice to say I assisted in my parents premature greying and balding. As a parent, I now understand their panic, but back then I didn't have a clue.

Then at age eight, Mother Nature cruelly intruded and presented me with breasts and hormones. By nine I was fully menstrual and in full pubescent swing, complete with mood swings and temper tantrums. How does one explain all this to an already brain-damaged nine-year-old with behavioral issues? My poor mother tried the bird nest analogy and I cried thinking I had sticks and grass inside me. I knew they would hurt coming out and didn't look forward to that! We sorted that one out together but I couldn't make heads or tails of what I was feeling. All of a sudden, the boys my age were really cute and very stupid. They made fun of my breasts and teased me incessantly. Older boys and even some men thought I was much older than I looked and flirted relentlessly. Many members of the male persuasion began to treat me differently and I just didn't get it. To make matters worse, my teacher at the time was a very strange woman who announced to the class that I was now menstrual and that I was not to be teased for it. The first time I went to the washroom, I remember four girls peering into the stall and asking all sorts of questions, none of which I had answers for. I was mortified and humiliated and kept to myself the rest of the year.

The boys teased me for having breasts and the girls hated me because they didn't. It was common place for me to be struck in the chest by either boy or girl during the course of the day and they seemed to get quite a kick out of it when it hurt as much as it did. Every little girl had gone home and told her mother that I had a bra and the next day every little girl had a training bra. I wanted to wear the cute little training bras but was already too big for them. My dad would tease and say he didn't know they had to be trained to develop and I would laugh at the other girls! Thank goodness for my Dads sense of humor!

It was such a contradictory time for me as I was feeling grown up sensations but had no idea what they were about. I looked like a young woman but was happy playing with my dolls one moment and trying to ride my brothers ten speed bicycle while wearing a tube top and cut-off shorts the next. I couldn't figure out who I was supposed to be and nothing was happening quickly. Like all children, I wanted to be a teenager now while the next minute I was happy being a child.

It was during these challenging preteen years that my brother's best friend picked me up on my way home from school. He was older than me, and like any little sister I suppose I had a little crush, so I felt grown up and important sitting in his car. He drove me home and followed me into the house saying he was going to wait for my brother to come home. He was being very nice to me which was strange because I was the uncool little sister of his buddy. The next thing I knew he grabbed me and pulled me down on the living room floor and started to grasp at my breasts and kissing me. I do remember crying and saying 'No!' and that his breath smelled foul. Suddenly my hero brother arrived and pulled him off me. I ran to my bedroom and cried while they were yelling at each other. I heard him telling my brother that I had started it and I didn't understand how. I never heard what my brother said to him or saw what happened. I was so afraid I was going to be in trouble that when my brother came to check on me, I begged him not to tell our parents and he agreed. It wasn't until a few years later that my brother finally told our parents when they pressed him why he and this person were no longer friends. I remember my mother was livid and wanted to go after him, but my brother, my dad and I convinced her it was over and done with. I don't know if she ever followed up but she was so supportive of me and my brother during it all. Although my brother and I were often antagonistic with each other, I was always proud he was my brother after that.

I remember one time when I was younger, my brother would walk me home sometimes from school. There was a big girl named 'Rhonda' who decided one day to pick on us on the way home. She was a bully and quite frankly I don't even remember what the issue was, but I do remember my brother out talking her to the point of her becoming confused and we walked away shaky but giggling. When it came right to it, he was my big brother and sometimes, I liked him. My brother and I are not close anymore and I take full responsibility for this being so. I regret not having a relationship with him and him being guarded with me, but this was entirely my doing. My brother often rescued me throughout my life, coming to pick me up and drive me home from wherever or whatever. I am sure it got more than tiresome and I know he had more than his fair share, but he was still there, always.

Teen Hell

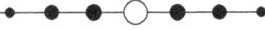

I BECAME SEXUALLY ACTIVE AFTER I began puberty, in that I was no stranger to masturbation. I knew enough to try to hide it but enjoyed the familiar sensations that went with it. I had my first voluntary sexual experience at age twelve and was frightened that I might be pregnant. I lived in fear until my period began and then came my first sigh of relief. That was to be my last experience until I was fourteen, but was also when my somewhat precarious mental stability came crashing down. I began dating and became overly sexually active all in a short period of time. The only good decision I made was to go on the birth control pill as I knew I did not want a baby. I am an advocate for birth control and when it comes to FASD, don't even bother with the discussions on abstinence, as we are reactionary creatures who jump in with both feet and do not think things through. As much as alcohol lowers one's inhibitions, it still has the same effect when paired with FASD. I was not about to stop being active and discovered I liked sex. It was familiar, pleasing and created a sense of power in my mind. Boys and even men wanted to be with me and I felt wanted, important and empowered. Of course, I couldn't begin to understand that it was shallow, empty and dangerous, I just knew it felt good.

My first real boyfriend was 'Geoff' and we would often sneak away from my swim team practice to a dance that was held at the same time in the basement of the 'Y'. We would kiss and cuddle but it never advanced past that. The next thing I knew I was hearing that he had gotten some other girl pregnant and I never saw him again until I was 16. I must admit I wasn't very pleasant with him and the meeting did not last long! I dated a few other boys and enjoyed the attention and experiences of dates. Soon I 'fell in love' for the first time when I was fourteen with yet another 'Artful Dodger'.

I was sure the world revolved around 'Steven' and was determined to make sure my world did. This boy was not the type my parents approved of, but initially they tried to be patient. When it became apparent, I was sexually active, the patience came to a screeching halt. I decided like many teenage girls that he was far more important to me and that I was in true love. We were going to last forever after all. We would sneak to his place at lunch time, have sex and be back at school in time for afternoon classes. We shared a love of guitar and music and often played love songs to each other, sure that this was how we felt about one another. In a few months when I learned he was seeing another girl the entire time he was with me; I lost touch with reality and went over the deep end. She was pregnant and expecting his child so I needed to be bigger and better than her.

Suddenly my world was about getting him back and I was prepared to do anything. Rejection had once again reared its ugly head in my life and it destroyed a little more of my sense of self. I decided being a damsel in distress was undeniably the only way to get him back so I began to hurt myself through cutting, drinking bleach and many other destructive acts. Still, I never felt any pain. I finally convinced him I was being abused at home and he became my avid supporter. Nothing could be further from the truth, but I had to explain the marks I had made on my own body. This accusation eventually involved the authorities and I had to explain it all. I accused my father of abusing me and caused such enormous hurt to my family (which I still feel tremendous guilt over). My father never hurt me in any way and was never anything but supportive of me. My brother has never forgiven me, but I know, amazingly, my father and mother have.

I began to see a Psychiatrist which was initially a great idea and was diagnosed with Post Traumatic Stress Disorder and FASD. I told him of some my experiences prior to being adopted, but never fully disclosed everything. I began to be able to manipulate him rather easily, thus losing all respect for him. It seemed like every time I spoke of my previous abuse; he became exited to hear more and more and this made me uneasy. By this time, my parents thought I might be better off attending a private school in Toronto, where the focus was on music, drama and dance. Although I didn't really want to go, I agreed and left the following September. I was sixteen years old.

I moved into a red brick, semi-detached house in the downtown annex area of Toronto, which served as the residence for the school. My bedroom I shared with another girl was on the top floor, facing the street. My roommate was from a wealthy family and she looked down her nose at me right from the beginning, so I was not off to a good start. She moved out after the first night and into a room with one of the other wealthy girls. I would travel on the sardine packed subway each morning to school and then home each night, to house parents who were not suited to the job. There were eight students in the house and two bathrooms, which made mornings unbelievably chaotic and I began spending time away from the residence, frequently going to the Metro Library.

The library was an enormous, magical environment for me and I found endless books on more topics than I could have ever imagined. I was like a kid in a literary candy store and I would spend hours there - staying until closing time, reading anything and everything from different countries in the world to psychology. I read on and believe I received more education from the library than the school. Millions of beautiful books, maps and pictures that I could endlessly disappear into and not face reality of any kind, my imagination was drunk with possibilities!

I would go home on weekends, but soon began to find reasons I could not go home, or would 'accidently' miss the train. I gained a new, older boyfriend who attended the school and who introduced me to the world of drugs and alcohol. We would spend hours smoking pot and having sex while looking forward to the next party. His father was a musician who travelled around the world doing concerts in the most exotic places. I admired all his art work and tribal antiquities in a drug induced stupor. My boyfriend introduced me to an entirely new world involving sex, parties, drugs and alcohol. At one of the parties he put together a party favor bowl literally the size of a salad bowl, filled halfway with just about every kind of pill imaginable. There were uppers, downers, Christmas trees, pink hearts, cocaine and acid, all for the taking with wine, beer or mixers. I loved my wine and chose pink hearts (uppers), and then proceeded to drink and smoke pot, hash and oil for the rest of the evening. I remember awakening in my own bed the next morning, still in my clothes from the night before. I had no idea how I got there and was also very aware I could not move. I laid there for a while thinking I was possibly paralyzed and was astounded that I wasn't dead and a little disappointed I wasn't. I resigned myself not to partake in the parties or the drugs any more as I was sufficiently frightened by my condition.

I became the loner at school and began to explore Toronto by myself. I went to museums, stores, art galleries and bars where I soon discovered if I dressed appropriately, I would not have to pay for any drinks. I was pretty, well- mannered and I could manipulate men easily. I met new people and became part of a new, older network, who assumed I was in my early twenties. I occasionally slept with older men who had no idea I was only sixteen. I never stayed around these people long enough for them to really get to know me and continued to go to school.

I adored this exciting life and experienced all sorts of people from stock-brokers to lawyers to musicians and artists. I attended parties with some elite and not so elite people, enjoying every walk of life and attaining a free pass everywhere I went. Sometimes I would go to these parties with my drama teacher from school who could easily be defined as a bohemian flake, most times I was on my own and no one from school or home had a clue what kind of life I led. I kept a locker at Union Station full of clothes to change into, mostly evening variety stuff depending on where I was planning to go. Thrift stores were perfect for finding appropriate attire for next to nothing and of course, I would never have to pay for my drinks or food. I would go to the station in my t-shirt and jeans, grab a few things from my locker and change in the bathroom, applying the correct make-up for wherever I was going. It was so much fun pretending to be someone else and I loved every second of it! I could be in the back of a limousine one night and on the back of a motorcycle the next. I could arrive with my date at someone's million-dollar home for a cocktail party then be in someone else's basement the next night, jamming with a bunch of musicians. If I knew where I was going for a party, I would often look the people up and learn what I could about them so I could fit in better, but if I went in cold, I pretended to be shy. I had the ability to con these people into thinking I was someone I wasn't and I was happier than I had been in a very long time. This was my year at school, until I met the boys next door.

The boys next door were all brothers and ranged in age from their late teens to early twenties and there were five of them all together. I chose the middle one, who was twenty-two, and began to flirt mercilessly, as I got to know the rest of the brothers. 'Tom' and I began a relationship that would last seven years and was the opportunity I needed to be able to leave home permanently. It wasn't so much that he was anything special, I was in love with the idea of being in love. I was also in love with the idea of being grown up, away from home and independent and that was not something I was going to wait for any longer. Subconsciously, I knew the people I partied with were just passing through my life and I needed someone I could manipulate over time in order to achieve what I wanted.

When school ended that year, I packed up and went back to my home town and began a summer job. I hated being home and losing all my new found freedom I had discovered in Toronto and began to devise ways of recapturing it. My old boyfriend from high school had come by my job with his baby son he had from the other girl, and proudly proclaimed it could have been my baby. I was genuinely disgusted and told him so in no uncertain terms! I decided I was beyond all this nonsense with him and I began flirting with a local police officer who came to see me at my job almost daily. He was a handsome, flirtatious, redhead and he thought I was cute. I decided one afternoon I was going to be with him and began to flirt mercilessly with him. We ended up getting together and spent the afternoon together. I was sixteen and knew everything of course and saw nothing wrong with what we were doing. I was quite matter-of-fact about our activity together and when it was over, I nonchalantly got dressed and said thanks for the good time and left. I believe he was rather stunned that he didn't have a desperate little girl who now wanted a relationship with him. I know now he could have been arrested for what we did, but at the time I was simply having some fun and escaping for the afternoon. After my tryst, I decided I was going back to Toronto before I ended up killing my parents or myself. I was miserable and missed Toronto. I missed the freedom I had there and decided come hell or high water, I was going back.

In my mind I was serious about killing my family to the point that I had actually planned out their deaths, before I decided it was better to just run away. I had placed some of my clothes in garbage bags outside my bedroom window behind some cedar trees during all this, which my father had found and brought back in. They knew I was planning something, just not what. I was far more discreet after that and contacted an old friend from high school who owned his own car. He agreed to help me run away and we planned out all the details together. I contacted my old boyfriend 'Tom' in Toronto and asked if I could stay with him and he agreed. I let him know when I would be arriving and finalized my plans to leave.

On the day of my clandestine departure, my Dad drove me to work as usual, and then my friend picked me up and drove me back home to collect my things. I was sure we would get caught while I loaded his car with all my belongings, but we didn't. We were on the road within the hour and I felt excited, terrified and guilty all at once, but not enough to change my mind. We pulled off the highway at lunchtime and I called my father to let him know I was alright and not to look for me. I heard the sadness and disappointment in his voice as he desperately tried to talk me into coming home. It was the first time I ever hung up on my father and that bothered me the most, but I got back into my friends' car and kept going towards Toronto. I knew I couldn't go back, certainly not because of my parents, but because of myself. I was so unstable I knew I could have hurt myself or them and I still believe this even now. While I now believe, other options would have been much better, like hospitalization, I know at that time, I made the right choice to leave. I was just on the edge of sanity and could very easily have fallen off.

I arrived at Tom's parents place and my mother came looking for me later that day. Tom's Mother lied to her and said I wasn't there, and that same day I left with his father to go to their cottage up north. Tom was away in England and wouldn't be back for two weeks, so it was a good time for me to collect myself and get organized. I spent the days laying in the sun, fishing and swimming while my parents worried themselves sick about my whereabouts and safety. My mother kept trying to find me, but did not succeed or didn't let me know she had. Just before Tom came back from England, his father and I returned to Toronto, and Tom and I began our life together. I eventually reconnected with my parents and even went back home for visits and holidays, which were difficult at best but mostly strained.

When I turned eighteen, my mother gave me information about my biological family and I began looking in earnest to find them. I secretly envisioned that same silly fantasy of them being perfect and looking for their lost little princess. I had read a letter that my biological sister had sent my mother, which included pictures of the family I had 'lost', and was amazed to see people who looked very much like me. I finally had similar physical features to a family and could see where I came from. It was very strange looking into the face of the woman who gave birth to me and seeing we had the same nose, hair color and eyes. We both had freckles and were petite women. I was excited at the idea of finally knowing who I was and where I came from. All my unanswered questions would be answered and I would finally belong somewhere and become 'unrejected', or so I thought.

I eventually made contact with a biological relative and made arrangements to go and meet the family. When the day finally arrived, I dressed up in the nicest outfit I owned and I boarded the train alone. I spent the entire trip there fantasizing how it would unfold, dreaming of falling into this woman's arms and her crying about finally having her baby returned. It was so far from the truth that I had no way of preparing for the bizarre reality that awaited me.

As soon as I got off the train, I spotted her. She looked exactly like an older version of me. This was 'Lisa' my 'mother', a pretty young woman in stiletto heels, hugging me and telling me how much she loved and missed me. I said nothing in return to her, I just couldn't say anything. The first part of my dream had come true but it didn't quite feel right, not like I thought it would. My intuition was tingling as I walked to her car with her, I couldn't understand why I didn't trust her. I tried to brush it off as she chattered endlessly during the entire drive back to her place, though I didn't hear much of what she said. When we finally arrived at a little white house in the country, there was a crowd of people waiting; I was so overwhelmed, I didn't hear any of their names. I was introduced to a brother, then 'Lisa's' fiancé, an Aunt and a grandmother as well as a mess of dirty faced kids who were apparently cousins, nieces and nephews. There were others there as well, but I honestly can't remember who they were, only that I was extremely uncomfortable and suddenly wanted to go home. All these people were flooding me with questions about my life and how it had been, who my adopted family were and that they must be very rich, or so they had heard. Thankfully, I told them very little and played the shy card which got me out of answering most of their demanding questions. I found them to be extremely pushy and brash, not at all the way I was raised and suddenly for the first time I found myself proud of my upbringing. It was strange to be surrounded by 'family' and find myself thinking of my parents and suddenly wishing they were there with me. My mom would have known how to handle these strangers far better than I did. I missed her terribly then, for the first time in a very long time.

'Lisa' was drinking immediately upon our arrival and after a short while, insisted we go to meet another one of my siblings. As 'Lisa' drove, I wondered where we were going in such a mad rush, as her driving was quite aggressive as though on our way to an emergency. I wondered what my sister was like as we drove onwards. She had gotten married quite young and had two children. My sister, her husband and children lived in a trailer park in the next little village down the road. After a short while, we pulled into a little driveway which seemed as though it was in the middle of nowhere, and I saw a tiny white mobile home. Out popped the family of four as though they were squeezed out of a toothpaste tube and again, I was in a vice-like hug. My sister was a taller, chubby woman who meant well but was ungainly and rather simple. Her children were dirty and her husband left so very much to be desired. He looked at me as though I was a juicy steak and I immediately felt dirty and disgusted. They invited us into her tiny home and we sat amongst dirt and clutter while her children screamed and played over a television that 'husband' watched while ignoring the commotion and eyeing me out of the corner of his eye. We spent a short while visiting when 'Lisa' decided we had to have girls' night out. So off we went again, 'Lisa', my sister and I were back on the road to wherever she decided to find the next drink.

We arrived at a bar 'Lisa' obviously frequented after another erratic ride and she immediately began drinking again. She chattered on about how she had been a good mother and come home one day to find that C.A.S. had 'broken into her home' and 'stolen me'. Of course, they had no right or reason to do this and gave her all the kids back, except for me. They kept me and she said she had 'fought them for years trying to get me back'. According to 'Lisa', she never gave away her rights and I had been adopted illegally. I knew this was a lie, but didn't say anything to the contrary. I had one glass of wine and my sister had a few mixed drinks while 'Lisa' pounded back shots and mixed drinks like she was dying of thirst in the middle of the Sahara. The drunken fabrications spewed out of her slurring mouth at me for a couple hours and I found myself disliking her more by every minute. She seemed to have a lie for every question and nothing was her fault, she had no sense of responsibility my parents had taught me and I found myself ashamed that she was related to me. 'Lisa' finally decided it was time to go home and began to gather herself and her belongings together. My sister suggested she should drive, but 'Lisa' lashed out with a sudden, unexpected vengeance and vehemently accused her of calling her a drunk, which she was. Instead of enduring further wrath my sister, obviously experienced with this behavior, looked at me and put her finger to her lips, nodding towards the car.

I didn't want to get into the car, but I had no idea where I was, how to get out of the situation or how to get back to Lisa's house. I crawled into the back seat and immediately began a panicked search for a seatbelt, before she raced away leaving a cloud of dust behind us. I immediately regretted my decision to get in the car as she drove weaving all over the road, incapable of driving a straight line, let alone walking one. I never prayed so desperately that a police officer would see us and pull us over, but it never happened. She dropped my sister off at her little trailer and we continued on our way back to her home. I never said a word the entire trip back as she babbled about how I had been stolen from her. We barely made it back to her place and she hit the garbage can next to the mail box as she pulled into the driveway. I was so happy to get out of that car that I could have kissed the ground. I immediately excused myself and headed for bed while she settled down with her fiancé for a few more drinks. Eventually I could hear them stumbling up the stairs to bed. I quietly cried myself to sleep that night thinking of all the excuses and lies she had told me during the previous few hours. She still loved me, she wanted to be my mom again, she never stopped looking for me, and she had never hurt me. Every word she had spoken was a lie and she was a raging alcoholic, still after all these years. She had not learned a damned thing with my removal and blamed everyone else for her pathetic drunken life. I knew I would never trust this woman much less have any further contact with her as she had spent the evening in effect rejecting me again, in favor of her first true love; alcohol.

The next morning, I was the first to get out of bed and I sat outside in the cold fog of the morning, watching the sun come up. I went through the previous night's events and tried to make sense of it all, to no avail. My sister soon arrived later on and we went for a walk before anyone else got up. She told me the truth of my beginnings as we walked in the cool summer air. She explained that she was three when the Children's Aid Society came to remove me from the home. 'Lisa' was rarely ever home and had been missing for three days by that point, leaving me in my sister's care. My eldest sister was five years old and she and I were removed while the other children were given back to 'Lisa' for some unknown reason. Her boyfriend of the moment had decided it might be fun to put out his cigarettes on my arms and someone had seen the marks from this and called the police. When I was removed, I was wearing an old diaper, had several burns on my arms and was half starved. I became physically sick when she told me this and she continued on with the telling me of her reality. She had endured so much more than I with endless boyfriends parading through, drugs, alcoholism and abuse. I became angry and disgusted as I heard of her experiences and how my eldest sister blamed me for not being adopted with me. My eldest sister had gone on to live in institutions until she aged out of the system. She was now a grown woman with children, arrest records a mile long and a new warrant out. She was about to go back to prison for selling drugs and had made it clear when she heard of my return that if she ever saw me again, she would kill me, she hated me that much. It was completely understandable to me how she was so badly damaged after the life she had; I had and still have nothing but sympathy for her. I made up my mind to leave that day and go back home, I simply couldn't take anymore. I went inside to pack up my things and 'Lisa' got out of bed just as my taxi cab pulled into the laneway.

'Lisa' begged me not to go and I told her I had learned everything I needed to know. I also told her I was glad I had been taken from her and hoped never to see her again. I did go back one more time to see her after my daughter was born, with my husband, but we didn't stay long. She was unbelievably even more dysfunctional than the last time I had seen her and my patience and desire to know about this family was no longer there. I never saw her or any of my other 'family' again after that, I don't even know if she is still living. As for my biological father, I met a man everyone in the family, except for 'Lisa', insisted was the donor. He was somewhat better off than 'Lisa', but not by much. I have never looked back, nor do I ever intend to again.

As much as this experience devastated me, it was the best thing that could have happened with regards to my relationship with my real parents who adopted me. I labelled them my real parents after that visit, because I knew they raised me as parents should. They taught me about love, responsibility, they cared for me and I began to truly appreciate who they were and what they had gone through with me, especially after my own child was born. My parents and I have had a wonderful relationship and I would never even think of looking back to that mess I left. My concept of who 'Lisa' was supposed to be has died and I have buried her in a shallow, unmarked grave to be forgotten over time.

I lived with 'Tom' and his family for a few years and worked at various clothing shops, Mac Donald's and finally a veterinarian's office as an assistant. I loved working with the animals and even enjoyed doing the bathing of the animals. When Tom and I would briefly stop getting along I would move out on my own and did this a couple times, before we got married when I turned twenty-one. To say my relationship with my parents was strained during this time would be an extreme understatement and I did not help to improve upon it. My mother kept trying valiantly to maintain communication with me and even endured my marriage to Tom, even though both she and my dad hated the idea. I knew when I walked down the aisle with my father that it was a huge mistake, but I did it anyways.

I would not admit to myself or my parents that I was wrong. My husband was damaged and I knew it. He was clearly unable to have emotional attachments and no idea how to express feelings of any kind, let alone love. In so many ways he had the qualities of someone with a personality disorder; however, he was never diagnosed with anything. He was as emotionally immature, cold and distant as I was needy and this made for a doomed relationship from the very beginning.

In July when I was twenty-two years old, I became pregnant and was overjoyed at the idea. Though I was quite ill during my pregnancy, I gave birth almost a month early to a beautiful, healthy girl, weighing five pounds, two ounces. My husband was devastated I had not delivered a boy and never showed any emotional attachment to our daughter or financial responsibility. When she developed severe Asthma, he was nowhere to be found for doctors' appointments or trips to the hospital. Finally, just before her first birthday, we separated and I was finally on my own with a sickly baby.

Once again, my parents stepped in to assist me in finding a new place for us to live. My mother and I scrubbed my new, one-bedroom apartment and my daughter and I moved in, ready to begin life anew. It was a dingy building with mostly immigrants in the gay section of Toronto and it was always a trial just walking down my hallway without at least one man making a pass at me.

I struggled for the next few years trying to hold down jobs; eventually losing them all, except for the odd dog obedience training. I had worked for a Law firm for two years gradually moving from receptionist to research and data processing. I worked as a Private Investigator for a few years before eventually going on social assistance and then to college to learn dental assisting. I graduated with honors and promptly moved my daughter and me further out of the Toronto area to where I was sure I would find a job.

My daughter was my entire world and I wanted to make sure she never had any hardship or abuse in her life. I tried to make sure no one ever hurt her the way they had hurt me. It was my mission in life to keep her safe and innocent, untouched and unharmed by anyone. I placed my daughter in daycare and found a new job working for a law firm as a receptionist. My ex-husband had my daughter every other weekend while I would party and enjoy myself. I did give myself two rules to live by; I never drank or partied around my daughter, and I never brought men home. I lived by these rules for her entire adolescence and never broke them once. I was not going to let anyone hurt her, including myself or lose my baby the way my maternal donor had. I was determined not to be like her. My daughter was beautiful and for the first time I knew I really truly loved someone. I made sure I never became frustrated so I couldn't hurt her when she was a baby, by placing a small stop sign over her crib. I doted on her, made sure she had the best I could give her and let her know every day that she was loved, I still do. I was fiercely protective, strict and the best parent I could be, teaching her manners and helping her every way I could think of. We are extremely close even now and I know she knows I love her more than anything. She is intelligent, beautiful, compassionate and an amazing woman now, who works with me every day in my company as my partner and Kennel Manager. I look at her now with amazement that we made it together her and I, we really grew up together. I finally learned how to be a child from her, she taught me so very much. She has taught me life skills I would not otherwise have. We are not best friends; we are Mother and Daughter who enjoy a closeness in each other's company in laughter and love. She knows I will always be there for her and I know the same of her!

Bartender, Bikers and Booze

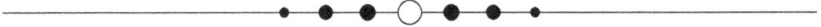

$$\bullet \quad \bullet \quad \bullet \quad \circ \quad \bullet \quad \bullet \quad \bullet$$

I FINALLY DECIDED TO MOVE from the Metro area when my daughter was five years old and establish a home in a smaller community in Southwestern Ontario. We arrived in our little community full of hope and promise, ready to begin a new life. I felt sure this was the right decision and change I needed to continue on my path. Here, I would find a new start, a new life and a new world of people. Perhaps had I been able to find a job in my chosen field, my life would have turned out differently, but I could not. I looked for months while on welfare and became disgusted with struggling every month just to pay the bills. I always made sure my daughter was well fed by living on rice and peas myself. I was desperate for work and began thinking about working as bartender in a night club. I had seen ads in the local paper repeatedly and decided I would look into it for myself. I went into a local club that looked promising, only to find out later it was the local biker hang out. I was hired first as a waitress and decided it was the perfect job for me. I could work evenings and yet be there to spend my days with my daughter. I hired a babysitter that I could trust for the evenings and it was another mother on welfare. I would pick up my daughter from school, and we would play together until dinner, then give her a bath and off to bed. The babysitter would come down after my daughter was in bed so I could go to work.

I found that I that I really enjoyed working at the club. I had two vastly different lives at the same time and I strictly made sure they never collided. I still had my first two rules; no drinking around my daughter; no bringing men home, and I would add one new rule to this list; no drugs ever! I am very proud to say very clearly, that I never broke any of these rules. My daughter never had to find me high or drunk and passed out, or with strange men in our home. I lived with two different named personalities and kept them very separate from each other. I saw my bartending as a play I would put on each night when I went to work. My bartender name was vastly different from my real name, and I would never show a trace of the real me at work. I aligned myself with the clean staff and patrons and began making respectable amounts of money. The acting I had learned in school was coming in handy and I was enjoying myself and the easy cash. I would go to work, do my job and go home.

I practiced with a new friend who had taken me under her wing and taught me to improve my drinks and pouring technique. She also protected me in the beginning by steering me away from bikers, letting them know I was not available, but more to the point teaching me how to deal with them. Bikers could be a very dangerous group if they set their sights on you. They would start out by being nice, then the next thing you knew, they owned you. The trick is to never owe a biker anything, not even a simple drink, as this was how they owned you and you would never stop paying them back. The owned girls were expected to bring in money, sell drugs, and be available at all times for sexual favors to the biker's club and prostitute, all in exchange for protection. I never saw the point in this and watched as these hardened, lifeless girls were beaten and some even disappeared. When a girl suddenly vanished and was labelled as 'on the road', we all knew what it really meant, but never spoke of it aloud. We found out after one girl 'left' that she apparently committed suicide by jumping off a balcony of an apartment building, according to the police. We knew better, we even knew who did the pushing but no one would ever say it out loud. If you were smart, you never became close friends with anyone and kept to yourself, which I did.

As for the drug side of the business, I have to say honestly it was easy for me to avoid them. I saw first-hand the effects it had on other girls', and that was enough to keep me clean. I would watch a beautiful new girl come in, who then became addicted to crack cocaine. Within a year, she would waste away to skin and bones, have terrible teeth and lose everything. I watched as many of them lost their children, homes etc. Eventually they all were diagnosed with hepatitis, AIDs or both and they all died, one by one. It was more than enough to keep me away from the drugs as I was determined that my children always came first in my life. I was determined that my children would never experience anything I had, including foster care and I made sure they never did.

Alcohol was a little harder to stay away from and on a few occasions, I found myself drinking too much, too easily. My children never saw me come home drunk because they were asleep and I made sure I was up with them every morning, headache or not. When I found myself drinking too much I would simply decide to stop and drink pop instead. The fear of losing my children was so great I was able to let that fear work in my favor.

The bar I worked in was unsavory, well known and very busy. I worked five or six nights a week and made a nice living. As result my daughter had the best of everything. I took great pride that she had private horseback riding lessons, swimming lessons and a wardrobe to envy. I was there every day to walk her to school and pick her up, cook her dinner and send her off to bed, all before I left for work. I had a babysitter there every night to make sure she was never alone and was well cared for. I was able to buy myself a nice car and maintained a two-bedroom apartment. I was still able to have my weekends alone when she went to her fathers for his visits and I took full advantage of them. Eventually, I moved us into a townhouse and had a nanny that lived with us full time. For the first time in my life, I believed I was in complete control and I was happy.

I was being paid to serve drinks and be friendly to the customers and I loved every second of it. For me, it was a game, a play I starred in and had a good run. I finally had a job that I was able to keep for almost nine years. I moved around and worked at different bars in the area after I earned my bartenders license. I know bartending for a living was not the best choice, but here it is simply; I maintained rules that I lived by and never became involved with people who could hurt me or use me. When I left the bar, the bartender persona stayed behind as well as the behavior. I think the girls who are 'owned and operated' by the bikers, gangs or the mob are definitely being used and abused, experiencing tremendous amounts of damage and as result have very difficult and often short lives. If you can stick to the rules that you work and live by, one can make a good living by keeping everything in perspective. I am the first one to say it's not easy, but it can be done, I did it. With the recession and years passed, I don't know if things have changed now, but back then it was possible.

I had a few short relationships with various men during this time, that I quickly became bored with and moved on. While I was not interested in a long-term relationship, I was able to recognize that I was not healthy emotionally. I knew I was unstable in terms of my past and my relationship with my family and decided to find another doctor to talk to. I finally ended up with a female psychiatrist who, through testing and therapy diagnosed me again with Fetal Alcohol Spectrum Disorder and Post Traumatic Stress. We talked at length about what I did for a living and she (my psychiatrist) felt I was doing remarkably well with the separating of real life and my fantasy life at work. She often encouraged me to leave the business, but never pressed it. My diagnosis did enrage me though and this time I was angry and felt cheated out of a 'normal' life. My life could have been so vastly different if this damage had not been done to me and I wanted to make my biological donor pay. I thought of shooting her or suing her but neither seemed viable let alone realistic. She never took responsibility for her drinking when I had been with her the two times we met and I decided to try to call her and talk about it. When I finally reached her, and explained my reason for calling, she became incensed and completely denied doing anything wrong saying 'Everybody drank and had perfectly healthy babies'… 'Everybody did it back then and there was nothing wrong' with me, according to her. She further told me to take responsibility for my own messed up life and not to blame her for my being a screw up. When I hung up the telephone I cried and hated her even more. I have not spoken to her since, nor ever desire to again.

'Hassim' came into my life just as I was thinking about finding 'Mr. Right' and settling down. I was almost thirty years old and ready for a change. 'Hassim' was a tall Middle Eastern man who told me everything I wanted and needed to hear. He was the perfect gentleman and treated me as royalty, in the beginning. Initially I thought I might love him, however it quickly changed when we moved in together. Slowly my life began to change and I was isolated from friends, family and the rest of the world. He began to control every aspect of my life and even when I was to become pregnant. I was soon expecting a baby and was completely cut off from everything and everyone. When exactly the abuse began, I am not sure, but it was gradual and slow at first. He was like every other violent partner, telling me how sorry he was afterwards and that it would never happen again. I was no slouch either and challenged him to hurt me, which he did. I felt so ashamed that I had allowed this to happen and yet felt stuck as I was unemployed with two children.

I delivered my beautiful, wonderful son when I was thirty-three years old. He weighed a whopping nine pounds and had a head of massive black curls. He was beautiful and I adored him with every ounce of my being. My daughter was proud of her new brother and he would laugh and coo at her in return. After my son's birth, the abuse from my partner became unbearable as well as the arguments. The arguments would progress to the point of threats and I called the police for assistance when he threatened to kill me. I believed that he would kill me and knew I needed help. When the police arrived, he was posturing and threatening to kill them as well. I finally had someone else to verify his behavior and promptly sent him packing. I endured months of threatening phone calls, stalking, and confrontation while trying to get my life back. One night I was awakened in the middle of the night and found him standing over my bed with baseball bat in hand. My daughter heard me scream and ran to the neighbors for help; we had practiced this drill many times in preparation. I was able to get to my son and leave the house with 'Hassim' following behind me. Once outside, the police arrived and took my statement. They found where he had broken into the basement and lowered himself into the house. They arrested 'Hassim' for trespass and suggested I move out of the home we had shared as under the law; he still had the right to be there as we had shared the home.

By the end of the next day, I had acquired a new home for my children and I to move into and I began packing. I hired a lawyer, filed for a restraining order and began the long legal process of gaining sole custody of my son. We moved in the middle of the night when I knew he was working a midnight shift and established supervised visitation at a local children's center, where Hassim's behavior was closely monitored. By the time we went to court, his case was entirely lost and I won full custody of our son, with his father having permanent supervised access only. Of course, this enraged him further and the threats of him taking our son to Lebanon began. I obtained an order forbidding Hassim from removing our son from the province without written consent from me, which as far as I was concerned, would never be given. I lived in terror knowing if he kidnapped my son, I would never see him again. This wreaked havoc on my mind and I constantly looked over my shoulder, waiting for someone from his extensive family to grab my son from me and run off. It never happened and eventually his father and I came to a point where we could be civil, but not after I had moved on and established a new relationship.

During the tumultuous time spent gaining custody of my son, I returned to the bar scene and worked as a bartender and worked with dogs on the side for extra money. I had given up much of my lifestyle years before, and had given up on bartending as well. I worked with dogs on the weekends and tried to earn enough money to support my little family. I had sworn off relationships, understandably, and was a bundle of nerves at best. I lived in fear most of the time and never stopped looking over my shoulder as my ex had a habit of following me everywhere.

I dated occasionally but did not have the patience anymore or the desire to play games with men. In the bar, I had many offers, but turned them down repeatedly. One man who came in would frequently talk to me of his family, work and friends and I began to look forward to his visits. We chatted over the next few years and became friends, disclosing tidbits about our children, relationships and humorous personal history. Shortly after Christmas in 1999, he came into the bar looking worn out and miserable. As we chatted, he disclosed that his wife had left him right before Christmas and he was devastated. He had been married to her for twenty-two years and was feeling absolutely shattered. We talked over the next few months and eventually he asked me to go on a date. My first reaction was an absolute 'No' but over time he wore me down. I finally agreed to a date, but then cancelled several times. I was terrified of this man, my potential feelings for him and my lack of trust in my own judgement.

I finally went on a date with him and it was the worst, most uneventful date I had ever experienced. We were both so nervous and wary that we simply couldn't relax and enjoy ourselves. The next time we saw each other we chatted and laughed about how difficult it had been. When he asked me out again, I said yes, but with ground rules. We would be friends with benefits only; no serious relationship or emotions were acceptable and he readily agreed. We both knew we were not looking for a relationship and yet needed companionship, and we naively thought this idea was possible.

For months, we dated by this arrangement happily and it worked, or so we thought. We would have our dates and then go our separate ways. The phone calls between us began to get more frequent and longer, and we began to talk every day. He would drop into the bar daily after work and I began to watch the door for his smiling face. When it happened, it took us completely by surprise and I was even angry with myself for letting it happen. After one of our dates, I kissed him goodbye and blurted out the dreaded phrase of death; "I love you". I promptly turned and ran. I left so quickly, shocked by what had just come from my mouth, he had had no time to respond. I yelled and cursed myself on my way home for saying such a stupid thing and was sure that was the last time I would ever see him. As I walked into my home, the telephone began ringing and I found myself dreading yet hoping it was him. I picked up the phone and said a timid "hello", then I heard him quietly say "I love you too, Babe."

I was very proud to say I had finally found the right man. It was due to incredible patience on his part, that we lasted almost twenty years. I learned so much from him and relied on his very being. I am often envious of his life, as he had a wonderful family right from the beginning of his life. He faced almost no adversity throughout his childhood, and because of him I have repaired my damaged relationship with my parents. He does not understand what I have experienced, but knows absolutely all of it.

I remember the day I decided to tell him everything about my past. We had since moved in together with his kids and mine and were desperately trying to make it work. He was having such difficulty understanding some of my responses and reactions to certain things that he finally asked me who had hurt me so very badly. We went for a walk down the quiet road we lived on in the country and I talked. During my talking, he would occasionally stop to cry or swear in rage, and I allowed him to do so without reproach. I kept myself emotionally detached, almost cold in my telling of the facts. I fully expected him to leave me after this, but he didn't. On occasion, he would try to hold my hand or hug me, but I couldn't let him touch me while I told him all my garbage. I was in a place where I could talk, nicely detached and that would have grounded me, brought me in touch with everything physically, it would have been my undoing. He stayed and showed more patience and love for me than I ever imagined possible. I still cringed a little when he got angry, half expecting him to hit me, but he never did. I trusted in this knowledge, where I never had been able to before. It is remarkable to me every day that this man loved me and I saw it in the little things he did and said. He was not a grandiose man who made absurd overtures, but instead was straightforward with a simple lovability that was his very being. What you saw was what you got with him, and there was no guessing required. He had a wonderful sense of humor; he could make me laugh at the drop of a hat and we laughed a lot. He teased me mercilessly and I loved every second of it. The best part was my parents understandably adored him. We had plans to grow old together and watch our children someday have children of their own. We also had plans to spoil our grandchildren to be, feed them chocolate and candy then send them home.

We ended up joining our two families to become one blended family and I love his sons as much as my own. He has three beautiful boys, all vastly different yet were fiercely protective of each other and their new brother and sister. They liked their new sister, although she was quite the enigma for them. This took time to develop and was rough and very difficult at times, but it succeeded. I adored his parents and I believed the feeling was finally mutual, although it was rather rocky at first as well. I understood their concerns with their son having been so hurt by his first wife, and tried to be as patient as I could. In the beginning, I found myself frequently reminding him and his mother that I was not his first wife and that I had no intention of ever hurting him, but this has long since ended. Convincing his parents of this took a bit longer but they loved my children as their own grandchildren and the feeling was most definitely returned.

My partner and I never got married, nor did we see any need to. We were more committed to each other every day and saw the ceremony as really quite unnecessary. He supported me through whims and dreams of owning my own business and helped me build it to what it is today. Without him, I am sure there would be no business or happiness for that matter. I initially began a training center for dogs with behavioral issues and also taught obedience classes.

During this time, I began to understand through watching my partner's sons, that my son was vastly different. As I began to reflect on his short life, I realized that he had drastically, suddenly changed at two years of age. He went from being a cuddly, happy baby who had started speaking full sentences, was almost completely potty trained and laughed the deepest belly laugh I have ever heard to a withdrawn, fussy child who back-stepped in speech and toileting. I never heard that beautiful laugh again or saw the sparkle in his eyes but instead saw fear and anger. As he got older, he became difficult to handle, would have incredible temper tantrums and was at times, even violent. He was also extremely destructive and his outbursts would last for what seemed an eternity. I took him to the doctor repeatedly and insisted that he be checked out properly, even though the doctor said there was nothing wrong. After many visits and finally a report from my sons' school, the doctor finally referred us to a Psychiatrist who performed many tests on him. When he was finished, he returned to his office where my son and I were waiting. This was the first time I heard the words "Not Otherwise Specified Autism Spectrum Disorder, Asperger's Syndrome and Pervasive Developmental Disorder". I felt my heart drop to my knees as I struggled to understand the full scope of what I was being told. I wanted to cry and shake the doctor, while telling him to fix my child, but there was no 'fixing' him. My son was now and forever more diagnosed as disabled.

Death of Perfection

THE IDEA OF MY PERFECT child or even the average, normal child was viciously struck down and I mourned the loss of him as though he had died. In a way, he had died and I was given a child with special needs in his place. I was thankful my relationship with my mother had been repaired to the point it had and I called her immediately for support. With her usual flair, she told me I had five minutes to yell, scream, rant, rave and cry, then it was time to start thinking about what my son needed. I will admit I took a bit more than five minutes and that night went outside and wept in the back yard under a bright moon. I swore at the Moon Goddess and accused her of screwing me over and not allowing me to have any happiness in my life. I sat there for quite a while when it finally occurred to me, that I did have an enormous amount of happiness in my life. I had two gorgeous, healthy children, three very brilliant, handsome stepsons, a man who loved me, parents who loved me and quite a nice comfortable life. What the hell was I complaining about really, a little extra work? I was ashamed with myself and immediately vowed to love and support my beautiful son, protect him and become Supermom!

As we worked our way through a forest of specialists, therapists and advice, I began to look at the possibility of a service dog for my son. I had heard of their existence and began to research the possibilities.

I found the cost was far beyond our means and decided to look into the training techniques and experience needed to train a dog myself. I passed the appropriate tests, and had over twenty years' experience working with dogs to certify that I could train a service dog and began looking for our first dog. My daughter and I rescued a puppy from a First Nations Reserve and brought the puppy home. Being a N.A.S.C.A.R. race fan, my partner promptly suggested the name Talladega, after his favorite race track and we shortened the name to 'Dega'. I began working with Dega and soon he became our very first service dog. He worked, ate and slept with my son, seven days a week and they were inseparable. My son loved his dog and as time went on and medications and therapies were added, his behavior steadily improved. Eventually his need for a service dog disappeared and he decided to donate his dog to a family with seven children.

After much discussion with my partner, I changed over my business to begin training service dogs and I invited my son to help me. He was only five years old, but was a very serious child and took the offer under advisement. I suggested that his job would entail taking care of any puppies we might have come to the center. After careful consideration, my son agreed with my proposal as long as he was my business partner and immediately began informing all who would listen about our partnership.

I set up my office in a separate room in our old house and set up desks for my business partner and me! We would have the occasional meetings and I would explain simple things to him such as how much food the dogs ate, or how many new clients we acquired that week. He was always very quick to understand how much money we could expect from each sale, but understanding overhead and expenses is still a very difficult concept to this day, even for me. Fortunately, I have my life partner and now my daughter to keep me grounded and as result our business has grown to the point where we own an entire training Centre.

My son graduated from High School with an 80% average and is a well-mannered, handsome young man. He still works with me occasionally, although he has given up the partnership in favor of video games. He has even been asked to give a couple speeches about service dogs. His communication skills have vastly improved as well as his people skills and he is able to accomplish more than we ever hoped for. His dreams of going to College and taking I.T. classes came true when he was accepted to college. We knew it would be a struggle for him and will likely take him twice as long to complete, but we also know he is more than capable, if just given the opportunity and time. He still has great difficulty in social settings and controlling his anxiety, but has learned that it is ok to ask me for assistance and does so regularly. He fights with depression and lets me know when it gets to be too much and off we go to the psychiatrist again. He used to dream of enlisting into military life but sadly understands that with his diagnosis, this is all but impossible. He is also a weather aficionado and knows more than anyone I know, about cloud formations and weather patterns. He is an avid Tornado hunter and dreams of chasing them across the country as I secretly hope against this idea.

He is my pride and joy and I am amazed by him every day as he accomplishes the little things that come so easily to others, yet are enormous feats of endurance for him. We have learned to celebrate the small accomplishments along the way, as even they are really quite monumental for him. We have celebrated shoe tying, buttons, zippers and haircuts with parties and cakes. Graduating from baths to showers was life altering while we cleaned up many a flood. His graduation from sleeping in a tent in his room to an actual bed, was celebrated with redecorating his room in a camouflage color scheme of greys, browns and blacks, although his bed still must be placed directly on the floor. His moving from a sleeping bag to actual bedding was celebrated with buying the camouflage bedding of his dreams. His learning of and maintaining responsibility and rules was celebrated with him being allowed to ride the lawnmower and even cut the grass, although we had lines everywhere and every which way. He is learning to cook and is now the head hamburger and hot dog chef in our household. And as he soars, I fly with pride right beside him, his biggest fan and supporter, encouraging and loving him as he reaches unimaginable heights. He is the most amazing person I know!

One day after watching a program on television about Veterans returning home with Post Traumatic Stress Disorder, my son turned to me and asked me if we could help. We had seen during the show how Americans were using service dogs for their Veterans and my beautiful son asked if we could do the same. I began looking into it the very next day. He was so excited about doing something for Veterans and as a family we decided we would charge a small fee to cover veterinary and food costs only, which would never change for the Veterans. At the same time, I began a war with Veterans Affairs to cover the cost of service dogs, which is just coming to an end almost twelve years later!

My son has experienced racism, religious persecution, violence and bigotry in his life due to the color of his skin and now suffers from PTSD as well as Religious Trauma disorder. With his father's family being Muslim, 9/11 and Isis, he lives in terror of being kidnapped and forced to join the 'revolution'. He is outwardly vocal against racism, injustice and religious zealots as well as those who harm women and children. He rages against those who commit atrocities against others yet still is a well-mannered young man with an amazing talent for writing. He struggles with depression, social confusion and control of his emotions yet meets everyone with a smile and a hearty handshake. He is the first to help a stranger in need and does so with great pride, class and grace. He is so much more than the man I dreamt of him becoming and I could not be more blessed.

F.A.S.D. Service Dog

⸻ • ● ● ○ ● ● • ⸻

WHAT EXACTLY CAN A SERVICE dog do for a child with FASD? Many children with FASD find it so much easier to love and accept animals, where they can't accept people. One minute they can be trying to hurt their parents or screaming in agony at their touch and in the next be gently stroking an animal and telling them everything is ok. The recognition of animal behavior is familiar on an instinctual level in themselves and therefore they can understand more readily what the animal is feeling. It is far more difficult for the FASD child to understand a person's facial expression, speech and tone than what a tail position means. Animal behavior is simplistic and uncomplicated, what you see is what you get. Human behavior is complicated, complex and can mean several different things at once as well as have hidden meanings, innuendos and motives. Most of the time we are guessing as children what a person really means or is trying to say, but we understand exactly that the dog is hungry or thirsty.

While service dogs are not for every child with FASD, there are determining factors that lend to it being a viable tool for your child. You as a parent will know how your child behaves around animals and will know if they have a calming effect on your child. If so, chances are favorable for a service dog fitting in to your child's world. If your child has ever shown violence towards an animal or is overly interested in dead animals, I would not suggest this route, a service dog will most likely not work and the risk to the animal is too great. I have also found in my years of experience that FASD children who also have a fascination with fire do not do well with service dogs. They often will try using bits of dog hair as a fire starter, not to mention again my desire to keep the dog safe.

Service dogs are trained with incredible obedience training to begin with, as well as specific tasks, like turning on lights, etc. They are then trained to recognize behaviors in the child that need to be disrupted and how to do so, such as head slapping/banging, or other types of self-harm. We have dogs that have been trained to accept facial tapping directly between the eyes for hours, but will interrupt skin picking on the child. The dog can also show an ability to know when a meltdown is about to occur and remove the child from the situation, by leading them. We know that dogs can smell the buildup of certain chemicals in the human body and alert to them, which is why dogs can alert to diabetes, epilepsy, cancer, etc. Dogs can also provide nightmare or night terror rescue by climbing on the child's bed at first noise or movement and provide deep pressure therapy by lying up against the child and pushing. Our dogs are also trained to lie down beside a child having a meltdown to encourage the child to sit so as to prevent self-injury.

We also teach the dogs to block flight or fight responses by standing between the child and another person, behind the child or simply laying down if the child runs. Sometimes they will run with the child, but keep them in a safe area by steering them away from potential danger as they run. Service dogs can also be used to redirect the child's behavior, for example if Johnny is becoming frustrated or over stimulated in school during an assignment, the teacher or Educational Assistant can suggest that Rover needs a cuddle because Rover is getting frustrated. Often times the child will self-recognize with this prompt and will respond" me too" and go to comfort the dog, which in itself comforts the child.

Service dogs can also be used for medication reminders by giving them a dog biscuit every time the child needs to take medication. Believe me once the routine is set, the dog does NOT forget its treat! As well, it teaches the child responsibility to feed, water and care for the dog, which in itself teaches the child compassion. If begun when the child is young, making a big deal over the task and saying how well the child does it gives them a sense of accomplishment.

If I had to, I'd say the bottom line is the dog can act as a secondary safety net, when the child's sense of safety is faulty. Dogs have an incredible sense of self preservation and will definitely pass this on to the child. They also provide the child with a friend who will be there no matter what and also help them make friends at school.

Having a service dog also identifies your child as having an invisible disability so people are less likely to judge or condemn a child during a meltdown, but instead offer assistance to the parent or care-giver. It also can prevent the child from being placed in restraints by police officers who think the child might be on drugs or other substances. Having a service dog is immediate rescue for an issue that might otherwise require assistance from first responders, lets the first responders know there is an issue and approach the scene differently at the outset. Let the police department know you have a special needs child that shouldn't be touched during a meltdown as it is physically painful. Let firefighters in your district know why your child will fight them from rescue because they are over stimulated and are terrified, as well as you having a service dog. Set up a neighborhood watch so if Johnny is doing something inappropriate, the neighbors know he has special needs and will respond gentler or differently. Let family and friends know this is brain damage and it cannot be cured, but is a lifetime diagnosis. The more people who know, the better chance your child has to make it through to adulthood without being arrested or trying to commit suicide.

When speaking at a conference where I am the center of attention when on the podium, I easily become anxious and overwhelmed so I take my service dog Oliver, with me. He is my best friend, my support and he has my back. He can remove me from any situation with the simple command of 'Out' or simply lean against me while I am talking to remind me, I am not alone. He goes everywhere with me and I am lost without him. Ollie takes much of the focus off me, has everyone admiring him, and he loves it! Due to physical conditions, I can sometimes lose my balance and he is always there to make sure I don't fall. He helps me up and down stairs, alerts me when someone is behind me and lets me know if someone is at the door. I am now hearing impaired and he knows this too, making me aware of the smoke alarm or other sounds I miss. He is the best one to tell my secrets to and he never judges me, we understand each other. He cuddles me when I cry and licks away my tears, but he also lets me know when I am being unreasonable. He gets this look on his face that tells me to step back and rethink. Most importantly, when I am unable to handle touch from anyone else, I can still cuddle with Ollie. It doesn't hurt, itch or is uncomfortable in any way, but is actually comforting.

When I begin working with a new client, they always meet Ollie first. He is my company ambassador, my business partner and safety net. Clients immediately fall in love with him and he puts them at ease so they can discuss extremely private details with me. Children who come to our Centre always ask where Ollie is first, then say hello to me. He works for cookies, doesn't argue and is always on time, although he does like to wander off occasionally. He comes when he's called, loves car rides and is always happy to see me. He is truly my best friend and I am already starting to miss him. Oliver is now almost nine years old and is semi-retired. I am currently training my new partner; Arlo and he is shaping up nicely.

Each morning I am greeted with a cacophony of yips, barks and howls as the dogs are let out from their evenings slumber. Each and every time I am reminded of a line from one of the Dracula movies where Dracula listens to the sound of wolves howling and says with a smile on his face 'Such sweet music they make'. To me all the noise is like music as it means the dogs are all healthy and happy. I will often go into the kennel early in the morning and the music will be playing loudly as usual. A favorite song will come on the radio and I will start dancing. I have one dog that starts dancing with me, as he jumps up and spins 'round. He is a white shepherd named Eochid, that is one of our white shepherd breeding studs and he seems to get such a kick out of dancing in circles with me. It is quite frankly the best part of my day and if it's a particularly bad day it is the greatest gift I could get! As I began to get into training service dogs, I felt like I had finally arrived or like I found where I belonged. I was in my comfort zone and felt like I was finally accomplishing something of value, that was needed.

Anyone who ever says to you that dogs do not have personalities has never owned a dog. I have comedians, philosophers, jokers and I have politicians all in the faces of my dogs. Each one learns at his or her own rate and we have our own Einstein's and a couple blockheads as well, but they all end up being wonderful service dogs! The dogs we rescue in particular are amazing as they each seem to know that they have literally been rescued from death row. They are so grateful that they work their little tails off learning as best they can and becoming some of the best service dogs we have working in the community. They are all thoroughly checked over by a veterinarian and temperament tested by us before they are even entered into our training program. Then, they go through many months of training and desensitization before becoming fully certified service dogs. When you put a service vest on a dog for the first time, they seem to know this is something quite special and the pride they show is incredible! They begin to look forward to having their vest on and to watch them pass a regular dog and see their tails go up and their noses held high with pride as if to say 'You can't do this and I'm more special than you!' makes me giggle each time!

As they learn perfect obedience followed by task training, they swell with pride even more as their confidence grows. They pass by dogs tied to poles and bicycle racks outside a store and they are allowed to go in, they start looking at the other dogs with sideways glances. The other dogs bark and pull on their leashes, but they remain perfectly behaved, not even acknowledging the other dog. In and out of restaurants, hotels, planes and trains while focused on their handlers with love and attention their handlers desperately require.

As my business grew and I became more known in the field, I soon became respected for my practices and dealing with the clients. People felt safe working with us in that we were not an American organization, or so big that they were lost track of. I always made it clear that I would not train 'cookie-cutter' dogs but train dogs to meet each individual need. We were a small family run business that gave personal service to each individual client and made them feel comfortable and relaxed. I have kept to this belief and business practice as many of these families have already been through the wringer and are somewhat 'lost' when they come to us in the first place.

We have trained dogs for Autism, F.A.S.D., Brain Injury and disease as well as little known syndromes that leave their children debilitated and without much happiness in their lives. They soon find a new best friend, positive attention and love in their new companions. Terminally ill children find love and friendship in a dog who gives them a few more months or years with absolute adoration. At times this job is either so frustrating making ends meet or painful upon hearing that another one of my children has died, that I just don't think I can do it anymore. Then I have parents who hug me and thank me at their child's funeral and tell me how happy their child was when they passed away with their dog at their side. Their gratitude is amazing during their grief and knowing that theirs and their child's suffering was eased just a little by a furry four-legged angel makes all the hurt and sadness melt away and I keep forging ahead.

I have seen the toughest soldiers wail with anger, while hearing their accounting of how he or she developed Operational Stress Injury. They can no longer leave their homes due to flashbacks and being unable to cope in public. Once they have their dog, they are able to become members of society, some have even become mentors to their fellow military family and done great things of their own, thanks to a little four-legged angel.

I have held many children and teenagers while they tell of their trauma and/or horrific abuse amidst heaving sobs. They have repeatedly tried to commit suicide because they can't live with the nightmares and the feelings of helplessness, as they try to cope. I've listened to their parents beg me to provide them with a dog as their last hope of keeping their children alive. I have also watched these same children and teenagers receive their dogs and go on to complete high school, then university and graduate with their angels crossing the stage with them to receive their certificate and degrees.

I have wept with Police Officers and Firefighters who grieve over the victims they couldn't save, who want more than anything to end their suffering. I wonder if I'm really making a difference. Then I hear how they are able to move on with their lives with their new service dogs, how they are finally able to sleep through the night without waking up screaming. I hear how they are able to repair or develop new relationships and then I receive birth announcements for new babies born into their families and how they enjoy life again with their new families and their service dogs.

I know the answer to the question of whether or not I make any difference. Yes, I am making a little difference every day, but the biggest difference is the difference the dogs make. The dogs are able to reach these damaged people on a level no human being can, basic instinct. The dogs automatically have their backs, just because they love their people and have the tools through training to know what they need and when. They watch their 'six' when others are standing too close for comfort, to lead them home when they can't remember during a panic attack where home is, to know when they are in a dis-associative episode their dog will keep them from walking into traffic or how the dog positioned itself between them and their gun during a suicidal episode. I have also heard how their dogs alert when their blood insulin is low or high, to alert them twenty minutes to an hour before they have a seizure. I have a dog that alerts to heart rhythm changes, and alerts when they occur so the parents can actually sleep in their own room together for the first time in years. The dog sleeps with her little girl every night and they often trade beds, I have the pictures as proof!

The best reward is all the pictures I receive from my clients with their happy smiling faces and a big goofy dog next to them grinning from ear to ear. I now have clients spanning the globe from England, to Brazil from Germany to California and in every province of Canada. Not all the dogs have been absolutely perfect and we have discovered some blips sometimes when they leave us, but we are still there to assist the clients with retraining or if severe enough, we replace the dog. Many of our clients have become like family and become pretty upset with me if they find I've been in their area without stopping by!

My business has led me around the world and I have become a lecturer, writer, advocate and expert in my field. Not bad for a kid that was supposed to go nowhere…when pigs fly etc. I now keep a little crystal pig with wings in my office to remind me of where I began and to keep me grounded. Of all the places I have been, my favorite place is still dancing in the kennel with Eochid early in the morning!

Death of My Father

———— • • • ○ • • • ————

I KNEW MY FATHER WASN'T well for quite a few years, but it never occurred to me that either of my parents were not immortal. As children, I don't believe we ever really consider our parents deaths as a reality until it approaches the horizon and we finally have to face facts. My father entered the hospital for what he knew was the final time, just after Christmas 2016. He had left his watch and wallet on his bedside table which was completely unlike him. He knew he was going to die and met death with the ease and dignity only my father could have. We had time to spend with him and say our goodbyes before he died and he knew, as did we, that there was much love to go around. Early in the morning of January 26, 2016 my brother called to tell me he was gone and I still answered him with shock in my voice. As much as I knew it was going to happen, I was still not ready to let him go and found it incredulous when it did. We prepared for the visitation at the funeral home and when I arrived, I prepared to see my father. I expected him to look like he always did and was shocked to see a frail unrecognizable man laying within the casket. The funeral home had done a terrible job preparing him and we were all so devastated that my mother ordered the coffin to be closed. I walked away crying to my partner that it wasn't my father in there and that I didn't know who that was. I went through the rest of the visitations, funeral and finally burial of his ashes, not accepting that my dad was gone. I could not and did not accept it until well over a year later, when one weekend I really needed to talk to him and it hit me when I went to pick up the phone and I didn't know where to call. I completely lost it and spent the weekend in bed sobbing.

I called my mother and all she could say was that it was about time and that she was happy for me that it was finally setting in. As well, my partner held me as I cried and he kept saying finally, but for me it was as though he had just died. It hurt more than any other pain I've ever known and still hurts to this day. I still cry thinking of him and even now am struggling to write this with dry eyes. He was our rock, our guide, our teacher and sometimes referee. He was a brilliant man and for me was the first man I ever trusted and one of the very few one's ever. He was an avid fisherman, baseball enthusiast and hockey watcher. He took enormous pride in the business I have built and often helped me develop new contraptions for the odd client who had unusual disabilities. He was always my go-to guy when I had a problem or diagnosis I couldn't understand. For my kids, he was an amazing grandfather who loved them and showed them so much pride. He was my son's biggest fan and supporter and let him know how proud he was of him. My son even read part of the eulogy at his funeral and everyone was so proud of the wonderful job he did. Until it came time to for my dad's burial, my mother asked my son to take care of the simple wooden box containing dad's ashes and bring it to the cemetery when it was time. My son watched over my dad for a few months and when the burial was arranged, brought the box to the cemetery with reverence and great care. Keir carried dad's ashes to the grave site withal the grace he could muster that day and as my mother wept, he protectively held her tightly. I could not have been prouder of my son that day, he was showing the man he was becoming and I knew dad would approve yet again. Our family dynamics changed drastically after dad died and my mother came to live close to us. As she approaches her 91st year, she too is becoming more fragile and I realize I am going to eventually have to face life without her as well and again, I am not ready. I need more time. I need forever, but I know this is not possible. We regularly go shopping, go for dinners and spend as much time as we can with mom and my daughter and son have luckily been able to be very close to her. I know the day is coming but I push it from my mind and hope I will handle it better than saying goodbye to my dad.

My mother has since moved in with me and my son is now on the tail end of college and doing well entering the world of computers. My daughter still works with me training dogs and helps bring our new puppies into the world. She is their second mother from birth and she loves each and every one. I am extremely proud of the individuals my children have become and know they will do well in this world. My partner and I have since separated and I am again alone on my journey. We are still friends and have managed to remain so, which I am proud of. I am looking forward to retirement and hope to write a few more books as I go along. This book has been a most difficult and challenging journey and I am relieved it's coming to an end. I have visited memories I did not wish to revisit and have laughed at others as well. I hope this narrative has helped, answered questions or given some kind of hope or direction to you as the reader. I cannot promise that your child will come through this diagnosis unscathed but I can promise it won't ever be dull!

Most of all when all this sounds like so much bullshit and you are wondering just how much more you and your child will have to face, just remember: you are all that is standing between this child who has brain damage and the rest of the world. One day they will turn around and not only understand, but mean it when they say…

Thanks Mom and Dad,
I love you too.

Final words

---•—●—●—○—●—●—•---

WHAT CAN I SHARE AFTER this long journey, about living with F.A.S.D. There is a difference between being a mother and mothering. To commit, nurture and raise a child with compassion, understanding and love is the real, most important part of the titles 'Mother and Father'! By the same token, it is important not to over-protect these children. While we do need to prevent bad decisions, it's important to let them many little decisions for themselves. They don't need to be life-altering and I recommend against this although they should be asked for their opinion, but smaller decisions like what color shirt is good for today.

Many families who have chosen to adopt a child with F.A.S.D. have made this commitment and should be supported by the community as a whole, instead of being judged for doing so. While C.A.S. have support groups and programs to assist in the rearing of these children, I believe it is important to also have programs in place for the children as well. There should be as much familial history and medical disclosure as possible so that you are informed of any other abuse that your new child might have experienced and I know that for the most part this is happening now. Realize that this is going to affect your child as well and seek help for them to be able to talk it through and realize they are not responsible for the behavior of their abusers. Remember the abuser puts responsibility on their victim and makes it their fault, 'If you didn't make me so mad', 'You need to learn' and 'Don't tell anyone or else'. These are huge burdens placed on a child and they may feel responsible for remaining siblings or be living in fear of the abuser returning. There needs to be a sense of safety and even a code word that you rehearse in case of trouble so that the child knows if they are afraid, you will protect them. As an abused child, I never knew this about my parents and wish someone had said 'I will protect you'. It was always assumed that I understood that, but I never did. When a child has experienced sexual, physical or emotional abuse, the damage is the same emotionally. They will see others as potential threats until proven otherwise.

There are many experts in the field who can assist the parents with daily issues, however I know the children have many unanswered questions as well, such as the biggest one of all 'Why me?' Unless the biological families are involved in the raising of the children, these questions remain largely unanswered. We are left to our own devices to imagine the answers and are usually way out in left field. I believe it would be useful to include a program for the children to discuss their biological beginnings and the effect, if any; it has or will have on each child. I personally know of one family who is struggling with this very question. The child's biological father is in jail and the child is acting out violently at times. He asks regularly what his father did to be in jail and he is asking if he is 'just like' his father. Is this the reason he behaves as he does due to a genetic factor passed down from his parents? While as adults we know this suggestion is nonsense, the child is struggling to understand his own behavior and lack of control. Does the apple fall far from the tree? I am the last person to believe I have the scientific knowledge to win a 'nature vs. nurture' debate, however I will add my own two cents. I believe 'nature' is responsible for the damage while it's up to 'nurture' to deal with the fallout. I believe behavior is learned by example and responses to this behavior. If a child throws a temper tantrum over a toy in a store and the parent buys the toy to shut the kid up, the child has learned a new behavior. 'Nature' was the one who told him to throw the tantrum, 'nurture' was the one who showed him it whether it pays off in the end or not. So, what is the bottom line; it is a choice we make whether or not to follow the behavior with a reward determining whether it will be repeated or not.

When I threw tantrums, it was almost always out of frustration and a lack of understanding. I was simply not able to put the pieces together in my brain and no matter how hard I tried; they would not fit. Instead of trying to come at the problem from a different angle, people would simply repeat what they were trying to teach. Now I approach things differently and if I don't understand something, I simply come at it from a different angle after taking a small break to relieve my frustration. I am frequently asking my mother or my partner to explain things to me and taking both their answers to work the final answer out. There are times when statements are made that I simply fail to understand and I come home and ask my partner what they meant by it. Most often, I have been paid a compliment and don't even realize it until he explains it to me.

While professionals might give you all the bad news and statistics, allow me to share some of the positive ones. Your child does not HAVE to wind up homeless, imprisoned or institutionalized. Some will require supports their entire lives, but others can have a successful life. Every little accomplishment will be monumental and hard earned, but can be achieved. Celebrate them like your child has won a Nobel Prize! Do not invite everyone you know for this celebration, keep it small and just within the immediate family, but still celebrate. Make your child's favorite meal or have a cake even, the bakery will write anything on your cake! Your child will display a talent for something, be it artistic, scholastic, sports etc. Enrich it and let him or her see their own ability and be proud of what they can do better than anyone else. Understand that there will be days of anxiety where they simply are unable to function and may need to stay home curled up under a blanket. Push them to be the best they can but know when to stop pushing.

As for school, do your best to get staff and administrators to learn about F.A.S.D. Supply them with pamphlets, books, information on seminars etc. Unfortunately, at this time, depending on where you are in Canada or the U.S., you might have to educate the educators and advocate ferociously for your child. If they refuse to work with you, find another school. I know it is simply said, however when I pushed hard enough and would not back down, they relented just to shut me up and make me go away. You are your child's only hope of receiving a proper education and you will most likely need to fight at some point for your child's needs. The teaching parameters or 'box' needs to be ignored, thrown away and forgotten about. I am not saying forget about your child going to school, I am saying forget about your child keeping up with everyone else. Focus on him or her alone and give them options, not demands. If they excel at art, use art to teach the rest of the subjects, if music, use music etc. Not all days were meant to be inside a classroom, but outside too. Not all projects must be written out, but can be acted out or sung. Do not push the child to frustration as that is when that proverbial switch is going to get stuck. Revisit another time and repeat, revisit, repeat.

As for your son or daughter, please have patience and don't give up. I have read many cries for help on Facebook pages for someone to help these parents and cry for them when they can't handle it anymore. But mostly I cry for the children who are then placed back into the system after having been rejected again and again. We have a great propensity for making bone-head decisions and fighting to the death for them, but instead of saying 'NO!' give options. The second we hear the word 'No' it becomes a challenge for us that we must pursue to the end of time. We can easily become fixated if given the chance and need to be regularly distracted. We may understand that we are

105

wrong about things but will fight to the death without understanding why or having the ability to stop. This is simply the damage our brain has and we cannot escape the loop without help.

When we become enraged, we must be removed from the situation. We cannot escape the rage unless we are placed in different surroundings away from what enraged us, be it a person, place or thing. We might babble incoherently for the first few minutes we are removed but it is far easier for us to regain control once removed. And for God's sake do not try to talk it out. We are not capable of discussion at this time, please call back later! This will only serve to refuel the rage and you will be right back to square one. You will not be able to discuss the incident until either they bring it up or days later when they are calm. We are not the kind of children who can sit down and be rational until far removed from the incident through time, space and place. I have wished constantly throughout my life that I had been able to say to anyone that I know everything I'm doing wrong. I know I should know better and it's most likely that I do, but I simply can't stop myself from doing. My switch is stuck! I've also wanted to scream that I know I am doing things wrong, is there anything I do right? People throughout my life have always been very quick to tell me I am wrong or doing the wrong things, but we so rarely hear what we are doing right. I know my parents praised me for my musical abilities and artistic abilities, but everyone else was so busy telling me I was stupid or that I wasn't learning the way everyone else was that the compliments got lost in the shuffle. Other times, I simply didn't believe I was that good; after all they were my parents and were supposed to be proud of me. Like any child or teenager, what my peers said to me meant more than what family said.

I had great difficulty making friends, let alone keeping them and was far more comfortable by myself. I am still very much a loner and prefer the quiet of home. Crowds of people cause me to panic and I don't care for loud noises. When I am in public, I can become anxious and frightened to the point of dizziness. I worry about what others think of me and am afraid of stuttering, which I occasionally do. I have learned I stutter most when I am becoming over stimulated and then quietly remove myself from the situation. When at a party, I will often walk around the room as though I am on my way to chat with someone and don't make eye contact or I will be busy serving food or cleaning up. If I keep busy, I won't have to talk to anyone or say more than a few words before moving on. If I do stop to chat with someone, I am constantly worried that I am slurring my speech, stuttering or that I sound stupid. So, I mostly listen, divert the conversation to my husband or parents or excuse myself as on my way somewhere. I am expert at focusing the attention elsewhere. With my hearing progressively becoming worse, I now mostly hear a hum when in crowded places. I can no longer pick out individual voices and this has led me to learn lip reading. When at a conference or speaking engagement, I will often ask someone to act as my translator for people I don't hear so that I can make it through a Q&A session. Initially I found this humiliating but have now come to accept it as a fact of life. I would rather communicate my message clearly rather than leave it undone.

Our business is doing well and we are constantly making improvements to our property, buildings and business. After adding Psychiatric service dogs to our company, I also began to include Brain Injury, Epilepsy and Disease, as well as Diabetes into our training programs. I have been quite successful providing very well-trained dogs to clients with many disorders who were desperate to regain control of their lives. When I began with the F.A.S.D. program it hit very close to home and I found that I still carried a great amount of anger towards my maternal donor. I cannot call her my mother, not only because she drank when she was pregnant with me, but because of the abuse I experienced due to her neglect and selfishness. Mostly I will not forgive her because of her denial of ever doing anything detrimental to me during pregnancy or after my birth. To me, a mother is the person who sees you through difficult times; supports you and loves you even when you're at your worst. I have a mother and a father who did not give birth to me, but are far more worthy of the titles than the people who did. They earned them each time I did well at something or behaved my worst, when I was the most ill and they did not desert me, or as I became successful and earned my achievements. They have the right to be called Mom and Dad, where my biological donors have none.

As a parent, I now understand the challenges and appreciate the hard work and sacrifice that goes with each child. The worry and fear that every parent feels when the child strikes out on their own for the first time and most definitely the incredible need to protect that child with everything you are and have. My biological donors never felt or did any of it with me, and continued to prove they were too self-involved to ever be a real parent. My maternal donors' choice to neglect and leave me as an infant in the care of two other children was extremely irresponsible at best. For her, everything was everyone else's fault; she never even attempted to accept any responsibility. The last time I saw her, she again risked my safety for her own needs. To me, this is not a mother, this is a selfish, narcissistic individual with no redeeming qualities, or at least none I want to search for again! It wasn't until I met my partner that I began to mend fences with my parents, so in all reality it took thirty years for me to grow up, understand and accept them. Will every child be this difficult, I suspect not all but some will?

My damage has been done and is still being discovered as I grow older. I am now moderately deaf; my joints are riddled with arthritis and my lungs are scarred by Tuberculosis. My memory has always been poor but now is made worse from the mini strokes I suffered several years ago, as result of a bout with the flu. I have had multiple surgeries to remove dying organs due to disease or scarring. My body still bears marks from cigarette burns, liquid burns and a leather strap. I am still prone to addiction, so I am extremely careful with alcohol, limiting myself each time I drink. I live in constant pain, but take no pain killers as I am too afraid of addiction. I have my own service dog who accompanies me almost everywhere I go. While the list of things I cannot do grows, the list of things I am learning is too. I have expanded my own world to include public speaking and writing, to educate the public about service dogs and F.A.S.D. Each time I give a speech it becomes a little easier to disclose that I have F.A.S.D. and I become a little less angry.

To say I have dealt with my past and have moved on would be dishonest not only to the reader, but mostly to me. I am dealing with it and probably will for the rest of my life. I still have nightmares that awaken me and I find that I have been crying in my sleep. Sometimes I still wake up hearing my own screams and I still occasionally become nauseous at breakfast. During the winter months, I still need to take medication for anxiety and depression and now for high blood pressure as well. I am however happier than I have ever been in my life, and this is an enormous statement in itself for me to be able to make.

I have learned to love and be loved; I understand that I no longer need to manipulate to survive. I know I am intelligent; I just need a few reminders now and then. I still am the world's worst housekeeper and have no real plans to try to improve that quality; I just hired a housekeeper instead. I also have terrible organizational skills and when I find my list, I will get right on that. I am the best mother I can possibly be and am extremely proud of my children. They are all healthy, respectful people and they all have good lives ahead of them. What have I truly lost in the grand scheme of life? Perhaps a few years due to ill health and stress, but I have gained so much more. People are capable and willing to love me, which I once believed impossible. But more than anything else, I like who I have become even though the journey here was appalling at times. I have had many great moments in my life and to dwell on the negative will only contribute to an early grave. What really matters now is that I can love, I can laugh and I can see the beauty in this world. I enjoy it every day as I finally find I am mostly comfortable with myself and I like me. Do I forgive and forget? Had my maternal donor accepted responsibility or just had a few drinks while unaware of pregnancy, then absolutely I could forgive. For me this is not the case and therefore I admit I am unforgiving and will remain so, unapologetically.

I have one dream left to accomplish for my personal bucket list and that is to see all alcohol marked with a 'Do Not Drink While Pregnant' label. It does not have to cover the entire bottle, but instead be a little logo that they use like the drunk driving labels. I would love to see laws changed to make it the mother's responsibility and punishable by imprisonment during pregnancy, but I am also realistic and know this will never happen, as it's against her rights. Smarten up people, the embryo needs rights too, to ensure a healthy beginning free from drugs and alcohol, but until it has a voice, no one will listen. Let's help people listen by pointing out the obvious, that it is unsafe for your baby to drink while pregnant. There are so many of us who can attest to living with this damage and how difficult it is. One little logo, it's a beginning to something much bigger and profound…a healthy infant.

For all the parents who have adopted FASD children, thank you. Thank you for choosing one of the most difficult roads, by helping one or more of my FASD siblings understand that they have potential, can know love, support and acceptance. We are all related under this terrible, preventable diagnosis and therefore unfortunately or fortunately, our family is enormous. You are not alone in this and there is help when you become overwhelmed. Do not try to 'keep it in the family' but seek out the assistance that is there. Accepting help is not failure; it really does take a community to raise a child with FASD. Maybe this community can help reduce the latest statistic of prisons where they have discovered that as many as 75% of the population has some form of FASD, FAE or FAS. I find this number shocking yet understandable and believable. Had these men and women had the supports that I had, maybe then the number would be less, but it all begins with disclosure. Without this, parents are doomed and the child faces a life sentence of misdiagnosis, mistreatment and most of all misunderstanding. Get as much information on your adopted child as possible and seek help from psychiatrists, psychologists and therapists. Pound on doors and harass people until someone listens.

If nothing else comes from this book, I do hope that the reader gains awareness and understanding as to the difficulties of this F.A.S.D. journey. Fortunately, the idea of institutionalizing special needs children is archaic but, I believe there is still so much room for improvement. It is my hope that this book in some way assists in recognition and the expansion of peoples understanding of just how damaging the misuse of alcohol and other chemicals during pregnancy can be. I still remember the fuss a pregnant woman made in the news recently about her rights being violated when she was refused service at a bar because she was obviously pregnant. Her apparent lack of concern for her unborn child hurt me so personally, because her child was about to live my life or worse and there was nothing I could do to stop or change the outcome, except to tell my story.

Resources

—————————— • ● ● ○ ● ● • ——————————

FASDcan

1. (support for families with children or adults with FASD across Canada)

2. http://groups.yahoo.com/group/fasdcan.

FASlink

3. (for individuals, parents, professionals who deal with FASD)

4. http://www.faslink.org/faslink.htm

FASD ONE

5. (for FASD Ontario Network of Expertise and Ontario FASD committees & coalitions)

6. http://list.web.net/lists/listinfo/fasd

FASDO

7. (support for Ontario families with children or adults who have FASD)

8. http://health.groups.yahoo.com/group/fasdo

Fas-bc

9. (FASD listserv for British Columbia run by Dr. Kimberly Kerns at University of Victoria)

10. https://lists.uvic.ca/mailman/listinfo/fas-bc

Justice

11. A great educational resource for families with children involved in the criminal justice system. Also, something to be share with your child's lawyer....

12. http://fasdjustice.ca/

Northern Family Health Society

13. British Columbia, Canada. Includes a myriad of publications and tip sheets for caring for people with FASD.

14. https://clbc.cioc.ca/record/CLB0506

Olderfas mail list

15. (support list for parents & mentors of adults with FASD)

16. http://www.come-over.to/Olderfas/

United States

17. **FASCETS**

18. (Fetal Alcohol Syndrome Consultation, Education and Training Services, Inc.) Providing an alternative paradigm for understanding behaviors.

19. Fascets.org

FASD Interventions Across the Lifespan

20. Perspectives on FASD Intervention: Research, News and Current Events (Canada)

21. https://fasdintervention.wordpress.com/

FASSTAR and FAS Community Resource Center.

22. Exhaustive collection of resources, training, and articles collected by Teresa Kellerman.

23. http://www.come-over.to/fasstar.com/

National Organization on Fetal Alcohol Syndrome.

24. United States. National FAS organization: includes multiple resources, support groups, publications, information.

25. http://www.nofas.org/

www.ingramcontent.com/pod-product-compliance
Lightning Source LLC
Chambersburg PA
CBHW022102020426
42335CB00012B/797